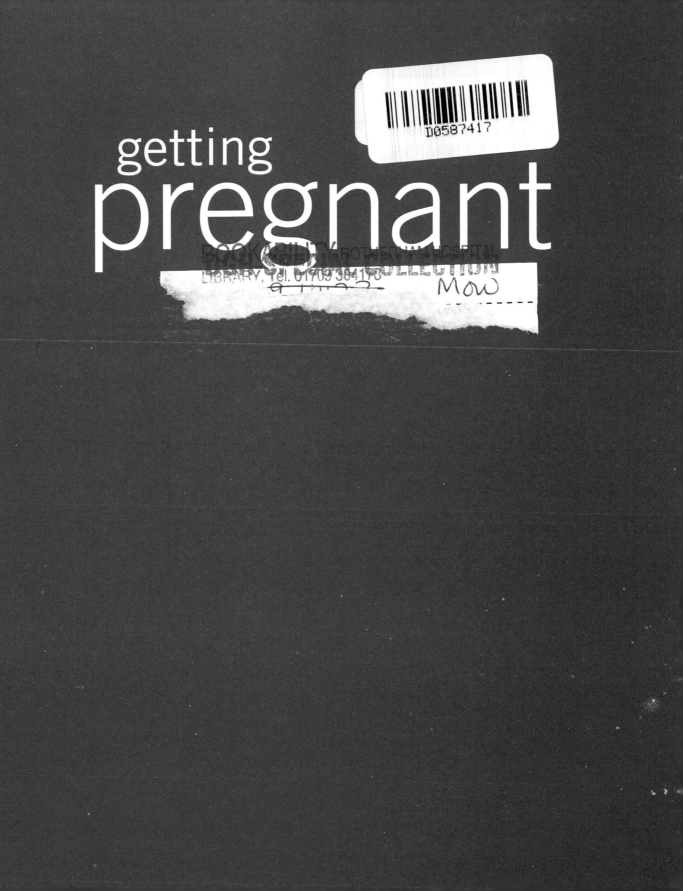

getting
pregnant

BOOK AVAILABLE IN: ROTHERHAM HOSPITAL
LIBRARY, Tel. 01709 304178
9/11/93
Mow

D0587417

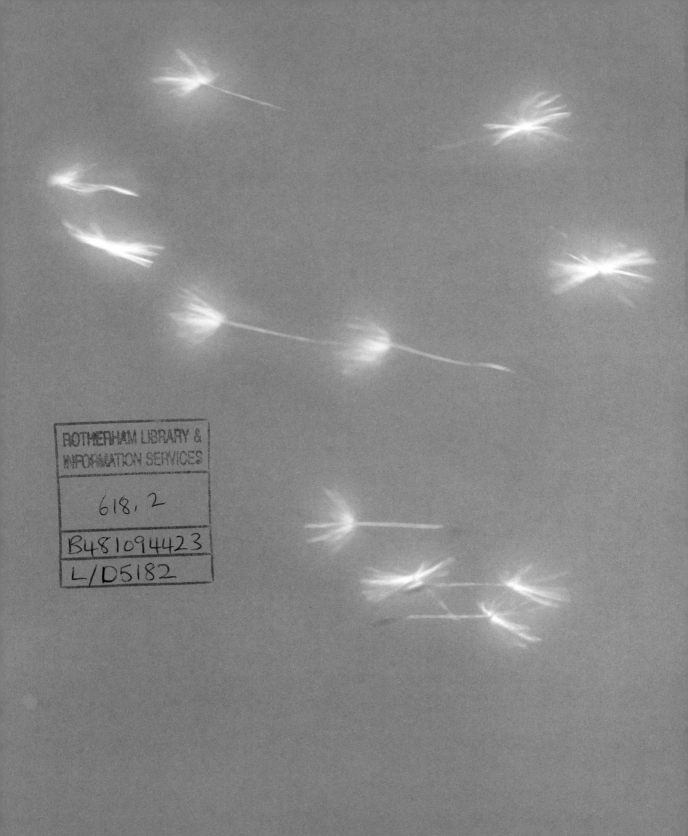

ROTHERHAM LIBRARY &
INFORMATION SERVICES

618. 2

B481094423

L/D5182

getting
pregnant

anne charlish

MITCHELL BEAZLEY

Getting Pregnant
Anne Charlish

Published in 2002 by Mitchell Beazley, an imprint of
Octopus Publishing Group Limited,
2–4 Heron Quays, London E14 4JP.

Text © Octopus Publishing Group Ltd
Design © Octopus Publishing Group Ltd

All rights reserved. No part of this publication may be reproduced or utilized
in any form by any means, electronic or mechanical, including photocopying,
recording or by any information storage and retrieval system, without prior
written permission of the publishers.

ISBN 1 84000 462 2
A CIP catalogue record for this book is available from the
British Library.

Executive Editors: Vivien Antwi, Lindsay Porter
Executive Art Editor: Christine Keilty
Project Editor: Michelle Bernard
Editor: Maxine McCaghy
Design: Louise Griffiths
Artworks: Kenny Grant, Peter Gerrish
Picture research: Jenny Faithfull, Rosie Garai
Production: Alix McCulloch
Proofreader: Laura Harper
Indexer: Diana LeCore

Typeset in Trade Gothic
Printed and bound by Toppan Printing Company in China

Contents

Foreword

Becoming pregnant and having a baby is a major aspiration of most couples, but for some it does not happen easily. This book is intended to smooth the rocky path when there are difficulties in conception.

Infertility is a disorder but not necessarily a disease. One of several disease processes may underlie it, but in many cases it is simply "unexplained". Modern lifestyle, diet, exercise, smoking, and a host of other environmental factors may play a role, therefore it is necessary to adopt a truly holistic approach when dealing with unexplained infertility.

Balance is key: avoid focusing on one single – usually unproven – alternative therapy, and instead give overall attention to a healthy diet and lifestyle. Modern medicine has much to offer but medical professionals do not work within a vacuum – by taking responsibility for your own health and well-being you will be giving yourself the best possible start, which will pay dividends. Confidence in medical care and the support of your doctor are also crucial, as it has been shown that the sequel to nothing more than a consultation with a caring, listening doctor may be a successful conception.

However, the longer story may be more problematic. The cycle of prolonged assisted conception is emotionally and financially draining, and the stress of clinic visits, drug treatments, and minor operations may be counterproductive. For this reason, good clinics should also offer counselling and, in some cases, complementary therapy treatments.

Anne Charlish's book explains and outlines the process of conception. Modern home testing for the fertile period is useful but it should not lead to an undue focus on timed, non-spontaneous intercourse. A basic appreciation that mid-cycle is the fertile time when periods are regular and normal should suffice. A change of environment on holiday, and relief from the stress of work and daily routine, is also beneficial. In addition, stopping smoking, stopping heavy drinking, and achieving your ideal body weight through exercise and healthy eating are all good starting points, and will lay good health foundations for the future. Everything that contributes to a successful conception also creates the best health for a successful pregnancy.

All these avenues are explored in this book, with both clarity and sensitivity. It is hoped that those reading it will find the advice and assistance they require.

Donald Gibb
Obstetrician and Gynaecologist
Hospital of St John and St Elizabeth
London

Introduction

This book is intended for everyone, female and male, who is intending to start a family.

There are a number of complex issues surrounding fertility and conception. This book explores each of those issues, and prepares both partners for the forthcoming pregnancy.

Preparing for pregnancy is largely a matter of ensuring that one's general health is as good as it can be – through eating good food, drinking at least eight glasses of water a day, regular exercise, and good sleep, as well as attending to any health and medical problems. Equally important is the need for relaxation, in which lifestyle and complementary therapies may play a significant part.

The impact of pre-conceptual health on you, your partner, and your baby, cannot be over-estimated. You will all be better able to cope with the demands of pregnancy, labour, and delivery, and the first year of your new baby's life, if you have each received the very best chance of good health.

Many people will wish to know how the woman's fertility cycle affects the chances of becoming pregnant, how often the couple should make love, and when are the best times for making love to ensure pregnancy without delay. This book covers these issues, but it also explains how to give yourself the best possible preparation for a healthy pregnancy.

It is not uncommon to experience a delay in conceiving. It takes many couples over a year of regular unprotected lovemaking. No one should assume that a delay of this length indicates that there is something amiss.

However, should the delay become prolonged, or should you suspect that something may be wrong or may be preventing you from conceiving, you should consult your family doctor with a view to referral to a consultant

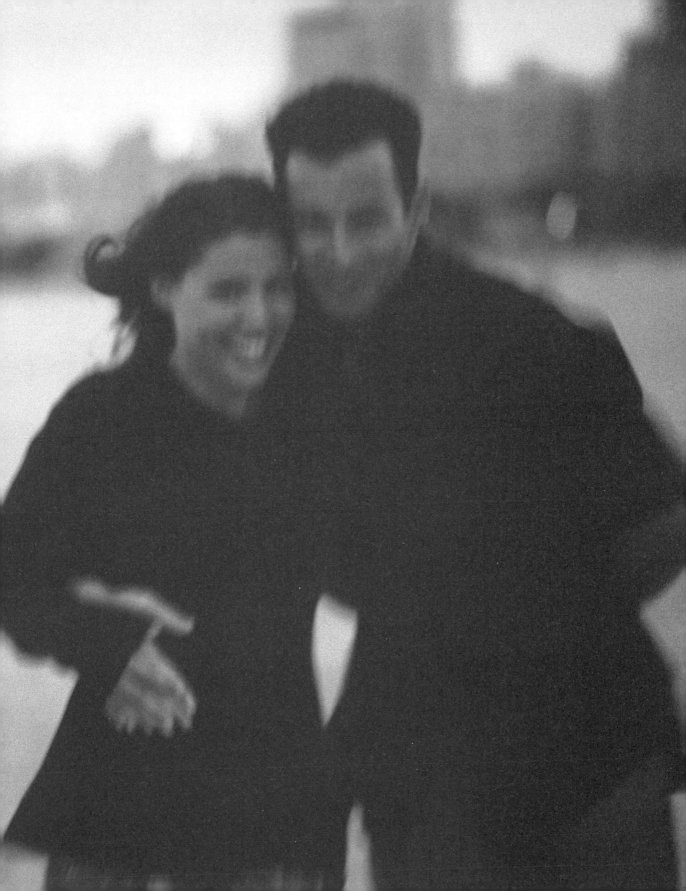

gynaecologist. If, for example, you have had more than three miscarriages, you should definitely see a consultant gynaecologist.

A minority of couples experience substantial fertility problems, and this can prove an extremely testing time. The possibility of infertility on either side represents a test, both for the relationship and for the emotional strength of both partners. Some people can accept delays and difficulties in becoming pregnant calmly, but others find the fear of infertility deeply distressing. As time goes by, they experience a roller-coaster of emotions, ranging from disbelief, despair, despondency, anger, frustration, and guilt, to a feeling of emptiness, a lack of fulfilment, and a sense of failure.

The woman's confidence may take a battering and she may feel emotionally exhausted as each passing month brings repeated disappointment. Waiting to see whether or not she has a period, or constantly anticipating her fertile period, may start to dominate her life.

She may at the same time feel astonished and angry that pregnancy does not happen easily and spontaneously, perhaps having spent many years using contraception to avoid becoming pregnant at the wrong time.

While I have been talking to people and researching this book, I have been struck by the bravery, patience, and stoicism of couples who have had to wait for many months, sometimes years, before achieving a pregnancy and the birth of a child.

Infertility for which there is no explanation even after many medical tests and investigations (known as unexplained infertility) is highly distressing. Yet couples who have had to accept that they are infertile and will never have a child sometimes find, to their astonishment, and perhaps as long as ten years after first trying for a baby, that a pregnancy occurs.

One couple in seven experiences delays in conception. It may easily take a year or more to become pregnant. Some couples do not conceive for two or more years, despite there being nothing amiss with either partner. Gynaecologists know of hundreds of cases of delayed conception in which, for no obvious reason, the problem resolves itself and the woman becomes pregnant. Sometimes there is no medical explanation for infertility and equally no explanation for why, suddenly, a successful pregnancy is achieved. So, although there may be moments of despair, it is worth remembering that there is always hope for the future.

There may be moments – or sometimes weeks – of distress and disappointment. Feelings of blame, rancour, guilt, and resentment may appear within the relationship. However, it is important that these feelings are acknowledged, addressed, and resolved by the partners and that they are not allowed to damage the relationship.

There are many straightforward reasons for not conceiving, many of which can be resolved with attention to lifestyle or with professional medical assistance. There are a number of medical procedures and investigations that can be carried out in order to establish what the problem may be, and these are described in the first chapter.

You will both want to do everything that you can to ensure a trouble-free pregnancy and optimum health for your new baby, whether you are lucky enough to become pregnant quickly or you experience delay in conception.

In addition to medical advice, this book will give you all the information you need about diet, exercise, sleep, stress reduction, and lifestyle in order to enjoy this wonderful event in your lives. By following this pre-conceptual plan, you may both feel better in health terms and happier in emotional terms than you have ever felt before.

Anne Charlish

Understanding your fertility

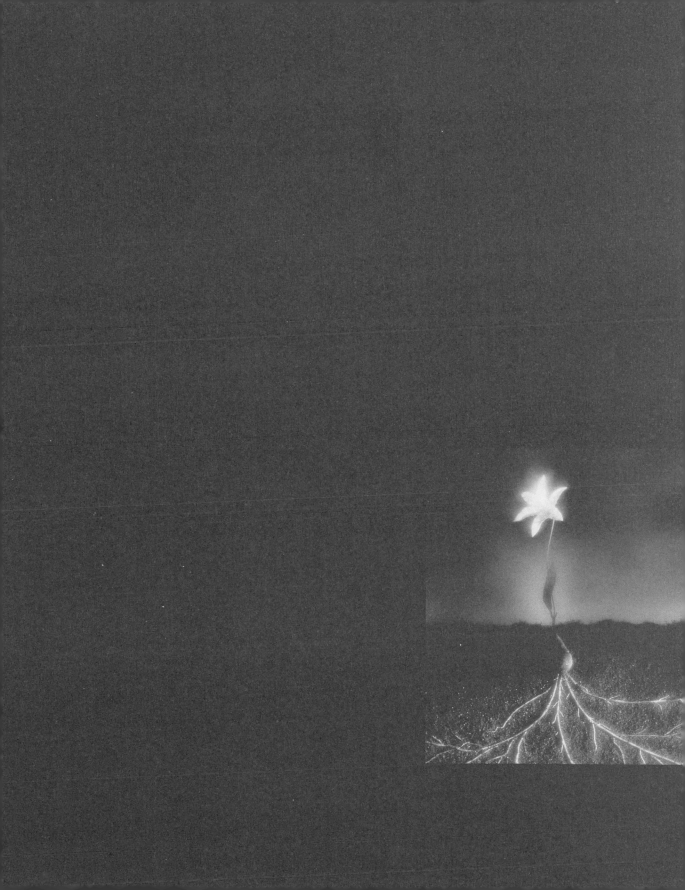

The female reproductive system

Having a baby is, for many couples, the most profoundly emotional and challenging experience of their entire lives. It is a time when both parents may pause to reassess their lives and to plan for a future that now seems to have more meaning than it ever did before. Planning for a baby, and for pregnancy, is a time of great optimism, but also a time, perhaps, for doubts about your ability, not merely as a parent but as an individual. These feelings are common to all prospective parents.

14

Conceiving a baby can sometimes take a long time. For many couples, the focus will for many years have been on NOT getting pregnant: it may come as a shock and a surprise to find that becoming pregnant is not going to be the automatic process you always imagined it would be.

For some people, getting pregnant happens easily without too much planning. Others, however, may have to wait several months, and you may need to give some thought to how you may best conceive and how you may maximize your chances of becoming pregnant.

Looking after yourself before attempting to conceive – known as pre-conceptual care – is of great importance, both for you as parents-to-be and for your new baby.

The egg's journey

A woman's reproductive system lies within the pelvis and comprises the reproductive organs: the ovaries, the Fallopian tubes, the uterus, the cervix, the vagina, and the vulva (see illustrations).

The ovaries are two glands encircled by the Fallopian tubes within the woman's pelvis, one on each side of the uterus. They are almond-shaped, solid, and greyish white in colour. The ovaries contain the woman's eggs.

When a baby girl is born, there may be as many as two to three million eggs in her ovaries but the number declines steadily from birth onwards. By the time the girl reaches puberty, only some 4–500,000 eggs remain. Of these, only some 4–500 (one every month or so), will

The female reproductive organs

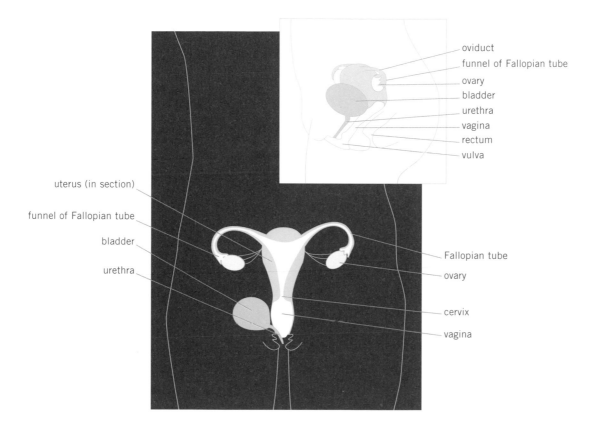

oviduct
funnel of Fallopian tube
ovary
bladder
urethra
vagina
rectum
vulva

uterus (in section)

funnel of Fallopian tube

bladder

urethra

Fallopian tube

ovary

cervix

vagina

15

be ovulated during the woman's adult life. The eggs are absolutely minute in size, as leading international infertility expert Professor (and Lord) Robert Winston explains: "Human eggs are very small indeed, about one-tenth of the size of the full stop at the end of this sentence".

The ovaries remain dormant during the woman's childhood. They start to function only at puberty, when menstruation begins. The menstrual cycle is also an ovulatory cycle, in that a woman produces an egg from one ovary each month, which allows the possibility of her becoming pregnant.

Each cycle begins with the first day of the period. A number of eggs begin to grow in the ovary until, after 14 days, one egg is sufficiently mature to be released from the ovary. This process is known as ovulation.

How conception happens

When it is released from the ovary, the egg enters the Fallopian tube. If it is destined to become fertilized, this will probably occur while it is in the middle section of the tube. It is during its journey through the Fallopian tube that the egg is fertilized.

If sexual intercourse has taken place without contraception, the man's sperm may fertilize the egg and the resulting embryo will implant into the lining of the uterus where it will develop as a conceptus, embryo, foetus and, eventually, as a baby.

At the time of ovulation, when the egg leaves the ovary, possibly on its way to be fertilized, it contains only 23 chromosomes: half the normal 46 chromosomes that all other adult cells comprise. The other 23 will be contributed by the sperm that fertilizes it. These chromosomes carry many thousands of genes that determine the genetic makeup of the baby, deciding its unique physical, mental, and emotional characteristics.

The menstrual cycle

During ovulation, the cells around the egg produce the hormone oestrogen. After ovulation, these cells produce a second hormone, progesterone, and together the two hormones stimulate the lining of the uterus to grow. The ovulated egg enters the Fallopian tube and travels towards the uterus. If the egg

has become fertilized, it will implant in the uterus. If it is not fertilized, it will not implant and, some 14 days after ovulation, the lining of the uterus, together with some blood, will be shed into the vagina. The entire cycle then begins again.

The shedding of the lining of the uterus is known as a period or menstruation. Most women have a period once a month, though the menstrual cycle may vary in length from 25 to 32 days each month.

If the woman is not menstruating, or is menstruating but is not producing eggs, conception is unlikely.

Female hormones

At the time of puberty, the pituitary gland in the brain starts to send messages to the ovaries to activate them.

It is not fully understood what activates the pituitary gland. The pituitary produces the hormones FSH (follicle stimulating hormone) and LH (luteinizing hormone). The production of these two hormones is crucial to pregnancy. FSH is responsible for stimulating the woman's eggs to become mature, while LH stimulates the follicle containing the mature egg to open and release it.

As FSH stimulates the follicle to grow to its maximum size, the cells that produce oestrogen increase in number and activity. As the cells increase, so does the production of oestrogen.

Eventually, oestrogen output is sufficiently high to produce a rise in the level of the hormone in the bloodstream. Once this happens, the rise in oestrogen in the blood stimulates the brain, alerting it to the fact that the follicle is now mature and ready to release a ripe egg. The hypothalamus sends a message to the pituitary gland, which responds by sending out LH. Within 36 hours after the rise of LH in the blood, ovulation occurs.

Immature eggs do not normally fertilize. If they do, an abnormal embryo may be produced which will be unable to survive or implant in the uterus. A mature egg contains chromosomes that have reached the right stage for further development. The mature egg is also capable of taking in a single sperm and denying entry to all other sperm. Furthermore, it is capable of ensuring that egg and sperm fuse successfully, producing an embryo that can develop.

This sequence of events is crucial to the understanding of fertility treatments: drugs that are given in order to encourage ovulation must be given in the right sequence, with the right timing, and the appropriate hormone tests. Otherwise, abnormal embryos may be produced, and these cannot lead to a successful pregnancy.

The female reproductive system is a complex and remarkable system, which, when in fully working order, can produce a pregnancy provided that the male reproductive system is also fully efficient (see pages 18–19).

WHAT MAY TEMPORARILY DISRUPT THE SYSTEM?

A woman's reproductive system can be affected by a variety of problems:

illness • fatigue • injury • very poor diet • heavy drinking • smoking • anatomical problems • sexually transmitted diseases

See also pages 26–41, where some of the more serious reasons for infertility are outlined. These factors may disrupt the female reproductive system but many of them can be resolved successfully with the help of medical and/or surgical intervention.

17

MAXIMIZING YOUR CHANCES OF CONCEIVING

Conception can easily take a year or more to achieve, but here are the optimum conditions for success.

- *Menstruating woman being between the ages of 20 and 34 and, ideally, between the ages of 20 and 25*
- *Man releasing healthy, motile sperm (see pages 18–19)*
- *Both partners being fit and healthy in terms of lifestyle, diet, and exercise*
- *Intercourse taking place at the appropriate time in the woman's menstrual cycle (see pages 20–25).*

The male reproductive system

A man's reproductive system comprises the penis, the testicles, the efferent ducts, the epididymis, and the vas deferens. Whereas women are born with eggs, men do not make sperm until they reach puberty. Sperm are made in the two testicles that are contained within the scrotum.

Thousands of microscopic tubes within the testicles connect to the efferent ducts. These lead into a single tube, the epididymis, which is part of the route through which sperm leave the man's body. It is about 12m (40ft) long, and finer than a piece of thread. At first, sperm cannot move on their own. The epididymis is responsible for transporting them, by means of muscular contractions within its wall. It also modifies the sperm, making them capable of fertilization. At this time, the sperm gain the ability to move (motility) by means of a process that is not yet fully understood.

The sperm pass through the vas deferens, which moves them past the seminal vesicles and the prostate gland, into the urethra. The urethra is the tube that connects the bladder to the outside world, through the penis. During ejaculation, the opening between the urethra and the bladder shuts, and semen containing sperm is rapidly transported along it.

During sexual intercourse, the sperm are transported in the semen into the woman's vagina and reproductive system, where they may or may not encounter a mature egg. When a sperm does meet a mature egg, fertilization may take place.

It takes only one sperm for a woman to get pregnant, but each time a man ejaculates, between 100 million and 300 million genetically unique sperm are propelled into the woman's vagina. It is just as well that so many are available because fertilization of the egg is far from assured.

So hazardous is the sperms' journey, that only some 200 make it as far as the woman's Fallopian tubes. Some sperm simply leak out of the woman's vagina, and it is believed that as few as 5 per cent get as far as the cervix.

The sperm have to be able to withstand the potentially hostile environments of the woman's vaginal secretions and cervical mucus, whose acidity protects against bacteria and potentially dangerous infections. Weak or damaged sperm simply won't make it.

Sperm cannot actually swim, although they are capable of some movement. They are transported by muscular contractions through

18

The male reproductive organs

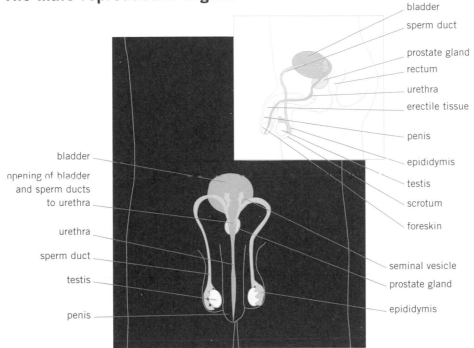

bladder
sperm duct
prostate gland
rectum
urethra
erectile tissue
penis
epididymis
testis
scrotum
foreskin
seminal vesicle
prostate gland
epididymis

bladder
opening of bladder
and sperm ducts
to urethra
urethra
sperm duct
testis
penis

the man's reproductive system and, when they enter, or are propelled into the woman's reproductive system, they continue to be transported under their own power.

The woman's cervical mucus is usually thin and watery, and capable of being penetrated by sperm at around the time of ovulation. Each sperm undergoes capacitation, in which the sperm cap is removed. Once this has occurred – and the process is not yet fully understood – the sperm is capable of penetrating an egg. Now the fertilized egg (conceptus) can pass through into the Fallopian tubes and the uterus.

Sperm can survive for perhaps up to 48 hours. Even if no mature egg awaits the arrival of sperm, an egg may be produced some time after they have arrived, enabling fertilization at that point.

Fertilization of the woman's egg may take up to 24 hours. Seven days later, the fertilized egg, having undergone a series of very complex changes, will become implanted in the lining of the woman's uterus.

Implantation of the fertilized egg into the wall of the woman's uterus is regarded as the moment of conception.

The best time to conceive

The only time to conceive a baby is around the time of ovulation, which occurs roughly midway through the menstrual cycle. So in order to maximize your chance of success, it is useful to work out when your fertile period is likely to be.

The sequence of events leading to the establishment of a pregnancy is ovulation, fertilization, and implantation. Ovulation is the release of an egg from the woman's ovary; the egg is then fertilized by the man's sperm; and if the egg is successfully fertilized it will become implanted, normally in the lining of the uterus. Fertilization by the man's sperm usually occurs within 48 hours of the woman ovulating.

It can be difficult to pinpoint the time of conception, because a woman's periods can be very irregular. Although it is known that implantation occurs some seven days after fertilization and that fertilization takes place within 48 hours of the woman ovulating, it is not always possible to calculate when ovulation itself occurred.

Ovulation takes place 14 days before the expected next period. However, in most cases this is not the same as saying it takes place 14 days after the last period because women's menstrual cycles vary in length considerably. They can sometimes be as short as 21 days or as long as 38 days rather than the average 28-day cycle.

Your fertile period

There are a number of ways in which you can find out when ovulation is likely to occur:

- If you have a regular monthly cycle, you will know when your next period is likely to start and from that date you can count back 14 days. This is the day on which you are likely to conceive. Even with a regular cycle, working out what is likely to be your fertile period means keeping a record of your periods for some months, perhaps up to a year, in order to establish the normal length of your cycle.

- If your periods are irregular, you may still be able to establish the day of ovulation. While calculations will not be possible, you will be able to observe changes in your body temperature and cervical mucus. Just before ovulation, the mucus secreted by glands in the lining of the cervix increases in quantity and becomes thinner. It also becomes more elastic, jelly-like, and transparent – a drop can be stretched into a long strand without breaking. After ovulation, the mucus again

The menstrual cycle

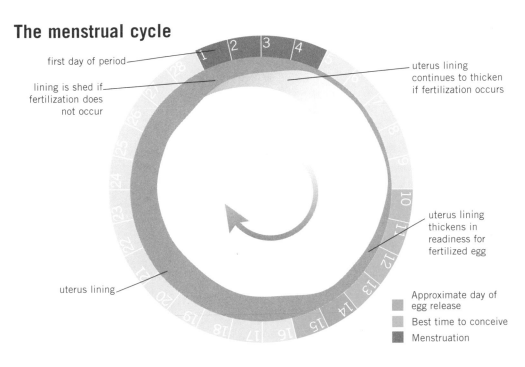

first day of period — 1 2 3 4

lining is shed if fertilization does not occur

uterus lining continues to thicken if fertilization occurs

uterus lining thickens in readiness for fertilized egg

uterus lining

Approximate day of egg release

Best time to conceive

Menstruation

21

The fertile period

Couples intending to conceive should have sexual intercourse within four days before ovulation, and up to 24 hours afterwards. In order to maximize the male sperm count and semen volume, some research suggests that the man should not ejaculate for at least a week before the woman's most fertile period. Other research suggests having sex at least every two days throughout the menstrual cycle to maintain a constant presence of sperm to await the ripened egg.

If your monthly cycle is regular, you can find out the day on which you are likely to conceive by counting back 14 days from when your next period is likely to start. To work out what is your fertile period, you should keep a record of your periods for up to a year in order to establish the usual length of your cycle.

decreases in quantity and returns to a milky colour. Any infection, however, may change the consistency of the mucus and produce a misleading result.

- You can also establish the day of ovulation by using one of the kits available, such as the Persona kit. These kits can be bought, without prescription, from your local pharmacy. The kit allows you to measure the amount of LH hormone that is being produced. This helps to establish when ovulation is about to occur. All you have to do is a simple urine test. A chemical will change colour if plenty of LH hormone is being produced. However, the tests are not fully reliable and can produce false positives. The kits are also expensive.

The reproductive hormones

Understanding the female hormonal cycle helps to pinpoint your fertile period – which is the only time you can conceive.

Hormones are chemical messengers. They are carried in the bloodstream and they are responsible for triggering activity in the different organs and parts of the body. The female reproductive hormones control the woman's monthly cycle and help to maintain the pregnancy, once it has started.

One of the ovaries releases an egg every month from puberty through to the menopause. The egg then travels along the Fallopian tube. If it becomes fertilized by a sperm, the egg implants in the lining of the uterus and a pregnancy begins. If the egg is not fertilized by a sperm, the lining of the uterus is shed and a period results two weeks after the egg was released by the ovary.

The menstrual cycle is controlled by the hormones FSH (follicle stimulating hormone) and LH (luteinizing hormone), which are released by the brain and which stimulate the ovaries to produce the female sex hormones: oestrogen and progesterone.

Variations in the levels of these hormones in the bloodstream determine when the ovary releases a mature egg, and they also prepare the lining of the uterus for a possible pregnancy each month.

If the egg is not fertilized, a fall in the level of the hormone progesterone occurs, and this causes a period.

- On the first day of the period (which is the beginning of the menstrual cycle), the hormone FSH is released from the pituitary gland in the brain.
- The FSH then stimulates a group of ovarian follicles to grow on the surface of the ovary.
- Over the next two weeks, which is the follicular phase of the cycle, the eggs grow and mature in the follicles. At the same time, the amount of oestrogen produced by the ovary continues to increase.
- As the oestrogen levels start to increase, the pituitary gland responds by decreasing its production of FSH. When the level of FSH has dropped, the production of LH is triggered.
- As the LH increases in production, the mature egg (usually there is only one) is released from the follicle in the ovary. This is the process known as ovulation. The mature egg now enters the Fallopian tube, where it may be fertilized.
- The empty follicle now changes into the corpus luteum, which produces the hormone progesterone. The corpus luteum

(the name literally means "yellow body") has only recently been understood and today research still continues about its precise function. It is an important structure, as not only does it produce the progesterone needed to prepare the uterus for a possible pregnancy, but its progesterone production is also essential for the earliest development of any embryo that forms following successful fertilization. It is known that if the corpus luteum is damaged in some way, an early pregnancy may miscarry. This second half of the menstrual cycle is known as the luteal phase.

- The fertilized egg travels down the Fallopian tube towards the uterus for the next 4–7 days. On the seventh day after fertilization, the egg starts to develop into an embryo. At this stage it develops floating tendrils (villi) of the chorion, which is the outer sac that will surround the growing baby. The villi enable the embryo to implant in the wall of the uterus.

- The chorionic villi now produce a hormone known as human chorionic gonadotrophin (HCG). Its function is to stimulate the corpus luteum to increase in size and produce more progesterone, which is essential in maintaining the pregnancy. HCG is the hormone that pregnancy testing kits have detected when they produce a positive result (see Testing for pregnancy, pages 142–53).

When should you have sex?

Some experts in the field of infertility are sceptical about concentrating too much on having sex during the period around ovulation. They do not recommend calculating the fertile period, monitoring body temperature changes, and using over-the-counter kits to find out exactly when it is happening.

It appears to be well established that the more often you make love without contraception, the better the chance you have of becoming pregnant. Statistically, the chances of becoming pregnant are in fact relatively low, but you can greatly increase your chances by making love every day during your fertile period.

Contrary to popular myth, making love every day does not produce weakened sperm, and there is really nothing to gain by abstaining from sex with the intention of producing more vigorous sperm.

One well-known study of conception rates seems to bear out this more relaxed approach. The results of the study showed that couples having sex once a month between the woman's periods took an average of 43 months in which to conceive. Couples having sex three times a month, had an average delay in conception of 15 months. If the couple made love ten times a month, the average delay was five months. Couples who had sex more than 15 times a month took, on average, just 3½ months in which to conceive a baby.

23

Stopping the pill

Most women resume periods within three months of ceasing to take the contraceptive pill. Just 1 per cent of women do not resume their periods within three months of stopping the pill, but some may do so later. If there have been menstrual irregularities before commencing the pill, these may recur after discontinuing.

Should you use an IUD/coil?

Some experts believe that it is wise not to fit an IUD/coil in women who have not had children. This is because of the increased chance of infection with this method of contraception. Such infections may cause damage to the woman's reproductive organs, notably the Fallopian tubes.

When is the best time for you?

There are a number of social and biological factors that you and your partner need to discuss in the timing of your pregnancy. Primarily, these include the woman's age (see pages 28–31).

From a purely biological view, the best time for a woman to conceive a baby is between the ages of 20 and 25. Biological infertility starts some ten years before the menopause (when periods stop or become irregular). Since a woman does not know when her menopause may start, and it starts earlier in some women than in others, it may be wise not to put off conceiving a baby if at all possible.

However, other important factors influence the timing of your pregnancy, including the stage that both partners have reached in their careers, their other responsibilities, whether or not they intend to move house in the near future, the state of their personal relationship, and their finances. All of these factors are important not only in themselves but also for the degree of stress or anxiety that they have the potential to cause.

Delay in becoming pregnant is often inexplicable but it is certain that emotional factors can play a part. It is also certain that any factors that may cause either partner any stress may also have an influence in the time that it takes to conceive. It may never be the perfect time to conceive a baby but there are times that are more right than others. For example, you probably would not want to become pregnant just as you were about to start a new job – it would be better to wait a while.

However, as fertility decreases with age, there may be a danger in delaying having a baby in favour of furthering your career, getting settled into the house you want, and sorting out the finances, for when you reach the time when you wish to conceive, it may not happen as quickly as you would like.

If both partners feel ready to have a baby, then that is the best time for you, irrespective of social and material concerns.

How soon will you conceive?

About one couple in seven experience some delay or problems in becoming pregnant. So this is not unusual, and it is nothing to worry about, provided that the delay lasts not much longer than one year.

About 90 per cent of couples achieve a pregnancy after one year. Another 5 per cent manage a pregnancy within two years of trying. Some of the remainder may succeed after trying for more than two years. Many couples who have been trying for a year or two to become pregnant are perfectly normal and healthy and have no fertility problems. Conceiving a baby sometimes takes time.

However, if you have not conceived after a year or so, and you are making love at least every other day during the woman's fertile period, you and your partner should consult your family doctor with a view to seeing a consultant gynaecologist. Ideally, both partners should attend all such consultations.

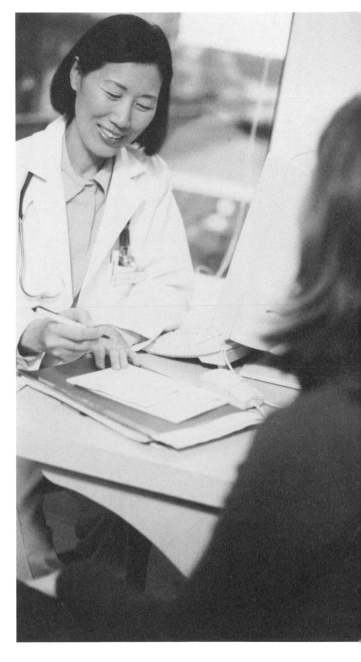

If you have been trying to conceive for a year or more and are worried that you have a problem with your fertility, you can ask your family doctor to refer you and your partner to a consultant gynaecologist.

The reasons for infertility

It is entirely normal for there to be a delay in becoming pregnant. Many couples experience a wait of some months between first trying for a baby and starting a pregnancy. This is nothing to worry about.

It is only when any delay becomes prolonged – more than a year, say – that you may wish to consult your family doctor. In the meantime, the best course is to have sex as often as possible during the woman's fertile period and for both partners to focus on all the aspects of their lifestyle with a view to achieving optimum health and vitality.

Are you dehydrated?

As part of your optimum health plan, you should be drinking enough water to maintain and repair all the body's systems, including the reproductive system. To avoid dehydration, which can lead to headache, tension, swollen ankles and a bloated stomach, you need to drink at least eight glasses of water a day – more if you also drink tea and coffee. This intake of liquid seems a lot, but after a few days your body will become accustomed to it.

In one-third of cases of difficulty conceiving, the problem lies with the woman having blocked Fallopian tubes. Tubal damage can sometimes be resolved surgically.

Are you getting enough sleep?

The body is renewed and reinvigorated by sleep during the night. It is at night that the billions of cells that make up the body are most quickly renewed. This renewal process does take place during the day but not so rapidly. Good quality regular sleep is essential for a healthy reproductive system.

As you are sleeping, the body's own natural cleansing system (the liver, kidneys, and

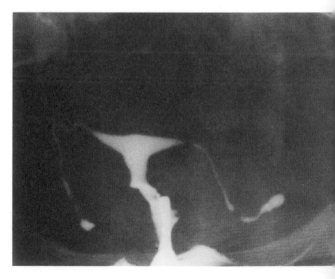

26

circulation) continues its work unimpeded by further onslaughts of toxins. Blood pressure decreases, stresses are relieved, and all the cells recharge and repair themselves.

If you don't get enough sleep, you wake up feeling tired, sluggish, and bleary. Your eyes feel dry, your skin is dry and itchy, your legs ache, and you feel shivery, apathetic, and unable to concentrate. Good, regular sleep is an essential feature of pre-conceptual care.

TIPS FOR GETTING A GOOD NIGHT'S SLEEP

- *Go to bed and get up at roughly the same time respectively each night and each morning*
- *Take no food or stimulants such as tea, coffee, alcohol, or nicotine for three hours before bedtime*
- *Sleep in a well-ventilated room (with a window open a little)*
- *Sleep in a room free of distractions such as computer, TV, newspapers, or work papers*
- *Sleep on a bed that gives you good support without being too hard*
- *Sleep in a quiet environment (use earplugs if necessary)*
- *Put off stimulating discussions (or rows) until the next day*
- *Don't make a cup of tea (which is a stimulant) if you cannot sleep*

GIVING YOURSELF A CHANCE

You can give yourself a head start by ensuring you're as fit as you can be. This means paying attention to your health. Make sure you're getting enough sleep and look at ways of reducing your stress by changing your lifestyle. Get plenty of exercise, ideally in the fresh air, give up smoking and cut down on your alcohol intake. Make sure your diet is healthy. Last, re-check your fertile period and discuss the situation with a consulting gynaecologist if you believe that you are having repeated early miscarriages.

27

YOUR GENERAL HEALTH

In assessing your general health, look at the following checklist in order to identify any problems:

aches and pains • allergy • apathy • asthma • bloating • constipation • cough (persistent) • dark circles under eyes • dental abscess • diarrhoea • feeling overtired, sluggish, tired in the morning, less zest for life • fluid retention (swollen ankles, swollen legs, swollen fingers) • indigestion • inflammations • irritable bowel syndrome • shortness of breath • swelling and pain in the joints

Consult your family doctor if you have any of these problems.

The implications of age

Biologically speaking, the ideal age to have a baby is between the years of 20 and 25. However, the biological aspect is only one of several to consider. Many women feel much more mature and much more able to cope with the demands of a new baby when they are older. They may be more financially secure, feel more settled, and be more prepared to invest the time needed to bring up a child. Many women are unwilling to start a family in their early twenties and they go on to have happy, healthy, normal babies in their late twenties or early thirties. Many women have also experienced the safe and successful delivery of healthy babies when in their late thirties and early forties.

28

Risk factors

Fertility undeniably decreases with increasing age and the risks to mother and baby become higher as the years go on.

Down's syndrome is a genetic disorder where both physical and mental impairment may exist. It can be inherited and it can also occur sporadically. The chances of a child being born with Down's syndrome increase with the mother's age. For example, the chance of a 20-year-old bearing a child so affected is one in 2000, while a 41-year-old woman has a chance of one in 100. (Older women are likely to be offered a test for Down's syndrome.)

The possibility of having a Down's syndrome baby may be the biggest worry of mature mothers but this is not the only consideration.

Other factors that are directly age-related include the increased possibility of:

- hypertension
- diabetes
- raised blood pressure
- reduced fertility in both partners
- both partners being less sexually active – when, as we have seen, conception depends on frequent and regular sexual intercourse
- the increased likelihood of an irregular menstrual cycle
- the increased risk of miscarriage and genetic defects
- problems with the woman's uterus (it may develop more fibrous tissue and less muscle with age)

The prospective mother of over 35 may also be more likely to experience:

- other general medical ailments that may have an impact on a fetus and that may need treating with medication
- generalized fatigue
- exhaustion during the process of labour
- fibroids
- miscarriage and stillbirth
- genetic defects
- babies of smaller birthweight – which may affect their ability to thrive

The older mother will naturally produce older eggs, and she is likely to have less vigorous blood flow and circulation (which could lead to poor nourishment for the unborn baby through placental insufficiency).

All these possible complications may seem very alarming to the woman over 35 who is expecting a baby or is hoping to become pregnant. However, you should not feel that you are embarking on a high-risk course. It is well worth remembering that 97 per cent of all pregnancies result in the safe and successful delivery of healthy babies.

Pregnancy can exacerbate any underlying medical condition through the increased burden it exerts upon the mother's body. There is an increased risk of developing or exacerbating the following conditions in mature mothers but they can also affect expectant mothers of any age.

Raised blood pressure

This is a particular worry during pregnancy as it may lead to a condition called pre-eclampsia, which is one of the most common causes of fetal death before labour starts (miscarriage or stillbirth). Pre-eclampsia is the precursor to the very serious condition known as eclampsia, which causes convulsions in pregnancy and can prove fatal. Pre-eclampsia is characterized by the development of high blood pressure, generalized swelling (face, ankles, wrists, and sometimes all over the body), and by the appearance of protein in the urine. Pre-eclampsia usually manifests itself at around 30–34 weeks of pregnancy but it can appear earlier or later.

Raised blood pressure can be controlled by lifestyle, particularly by paying attention to diet and weight gain. Smoking increases blood pressure, so if you smoke, give it up.

Diabetes

A pregnant woman who has established diabetes needs close medical supervision so that her blood sugar and insulin levels are carefully controlled. She may therefore expect to attend antenatal clinics more frequently than non-diabetic women and to have repeated blood and urine tests, so that any potential problem can be promptly identified and treated.

You can test your own blood sugar level at home using a special kit. Every diabetic woman will be positively encouraged to accept hospital antenatal care and a hospital delivery in order to ensure a successful birth. A home birth would present a high risk to the baby because of the lack of the facility to check and control the blood sugar.

Pregnancy diabetes is a form of the condition that occurs in pregnancy and clears up soon after the birth. It requires just as much monitoring as established diabetes and women who suffer from this disorder will need good antenatal care.

Antenatal care

All the conditions described above present a greater risk during pregnancy, but it is important to remember that with good antenatal care, risks can be identified promptly, monitored, and treated.

It is also well worth remembering that pregnancy is not an illness: antenatal care exists only in order to diagnose any potential problem well ahead of time.

Time

The last factor that women over 35 should consider is that if they experience any delay or difficulty with conception, it may take time to resolve. For instance, a 35-year-old who experiences delay in conceiving is likely to be over 36 by the time that fertility investigations begin (see pages 42–9). Should, for example, a laparoscopic investigation at the age of 36 or 37 show that she has blocked Fallopian tubes, it may take another few months to have this treated surgically and for her to recover, by which time she may be 38. During these years, her fertility, and that of her partner, is decreasing, and at the same time the possibility of general medical disorders is increasing.

For those couples who decide to undergo artificial insemination or assisted conception (see pages 132–41), time is now of the essence. These procedures can be very time-consuming and, ideally, they should be embarked upon earlier rather than later in the woman's childbearing years.

At the beginning of this section, it was noted that the ideal age at which to conceive a baby, biologically speaking, is between the years of 20 and 25. But what of the younger mother? The teenage mother's body may not be fully mature, she may not have completed her education, and she and her partner may not be emotionally mature and able to cope with the demands of having a baby and bringing up a child. So, although many women under the age of 20 have healthy babies, and bring them up very successfully, it may not be the ideal age, either medically or personally.

Looking after your health and choosing the time that feels right for you to have a baby are more important to a successful pregnancy than worrying about getting pregnant at the optimum age.

30

THE BIOLOGICAL CLOCK

*The implications of increasing age –
the biological clock – is an undeniably
important factor in deciding when you
and your partner would like to have a
baby. However, you must also feel that
the time is personally right for you.*

*Maturity, the sense of being in your
prime, a sense of knowing where you
are going in life, and a feeling that
you have established yourself in your
job are all important considerations in
your decision.*

*Above all, a strong, loving
relationship, in which there is total
trust and complete commitment, is
an essential factor in deciding that
you and your partner are ready to
start a baby.*

Maintaining a healthy weight

Being either underweight or overweight is potentially harmful to your general health and it can also undermine your chances of conceiving.

Female ballet dancers and athletes, who may be below their optimum weight, may find that their periods decrease in frequency or stop. They are – at least temporarily – infertile.

At the other end of the scale, women who are overweight may also experience delay or difficulty in conceiving, even though their periods may not have stopped. Being overweight is known to decrease fertility. It tends to make all the systems of the body function less effectively, and excess body fat is definitely associated with a failure to ovulate. The overweight male also has an increased chance of infertility. On the other hand, losing too much weight can also cause infertility.

Overweight women, when they have ovulatory problems, are much more difficult to treat and run greater risks from the results of treatment. The most notable health risks of being overweight, both when trying to become pregnant and while maintaining a pregnancy, are an increased tendency to high blood pressure, diabetes, and kidney disease.

While overweight women are less likely to conceive, if they do become pregnant they are more likely to suffer birth complications and

WHAT IS YOUR BODY MASS INDEX?

To help you determine your health rating, you can check out your Body Mass Index (BMI). To calculate this figure you need to know your weight in kilograms and your height in metres.

1 Convert your weight from lb to kg by dividing it by 2.2.
2 Convert your height from inches to metres by dividing it by 39.4, then square it.
3 Divide 1 by 2. This is your BMI.

For example, if your weight is 65kg, and height 1.68m, first multiply 1.68 x 1.68 = 2.82. Next, divide 65 by 2.82. Your BMI is 23.

A BMI of over 40 will adversely affect your fertility and is also a serious health risk. The ideal is a BMI of between 20 and 25. If it is over 30 you need to lose weight. If your BMI is under 20, concentrate on gaining weight by eating plenty of protein and carbohydrate, having a full breakfast, and a generous lunch and dinner.

are more likely to produce a stillborn child. All the general health risks associated with being overweight can have an impact on becoming pregnant.

Quality of life

Being just a little overweight in your twenties may not appear to be a very serious cause of worry. The problem comes later, perhaps in your thirties, when you discover that it is no longer as easy to shed that extra weight. By now, you may be just a little less active and your metabolism may have slowed a little with your age. In addition, you may have more money to spend on eating out, socializing, and alcohol – all of which help to pile on the calories. Once you are into your early forties, it is harder still to lose weight and easier than ever to gain it.

For parents-to-be, another significant risk of being overweight is that your chances of dying prematurely rise significantly with each extra stone you carry. If, for example, you weigh 83kg (13st) instead of the 64kg (10st) that would be ideal for your height and build, you are 30 per cent overweight and, more importantly, your chances of dying within a given period are increased by 60 per cent. (See Eating well and staying in shape, pages 62–117.)

Swimming regularly is the ideal way of maintaining a healthy, toned body, both before and during pregnancy. Swimming, combined with good diet, boosts the circulation and tones up the muscles.

IS YOUR HEALTH SUFFERING?

Many of us are overweight but still fortunate enough not to have developed any serious health risks. However, you may already have experienced warning signs, such as:

feeling overtired • shortness of breath • fluid retention (oedema) • aches and pains • swelling in the joints, especially in the hip and knee • back problems • less zest for life • problems with the feet such as collapsed arches, bunions • indigestion • headache • constipation

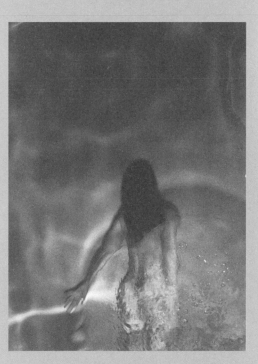

33

Sexual health check

A woman may not be aware that she has a sexually transmitted infection because there are sometimes no symptoms. However, if disorders of this kind remain untreated they can affect her general well-being as well as her fertility.

34

Pregnancy can sometimes exacerbate an underlying disorder not previously suspected, and treatment may be more complicated once pregnancy occurs. It is recommended that any woman, before attempting to conceive, should have a well-woman check, arranged through her family doctor, so that any of the following infectious conditions can be ruled out:

Bacterial infections: chlamydia, syphilis, and gonorrhoea, all of which can be cured with antibiotics

Viral infections: herpes, hepatitis, and HIV
Not all infections of the reproductive system are sexually transmitted. Tubal infections, which can cause temporary infertility, are sometimes caused by some other route. Any infection can damage the Fallopian tubes and thus reduce the risk of conceiving.

Of all the sexually transmitted diseases, chlamydia is the one clearly linked to infertility, but other STDs can damage the unborn child.

BE AWARE OF SYMPTOMS

Symptoms of sexually transmitted infection may include:

lower abdominal pain • pain during or after sex • bleeding after sex • irregular spotting or bleeding between periods • sudden onset of much heavier periods after starting a new relationship • pain on passing urine • increased or foul-smelling vaginal discharge • rash, spots, lumps, itching, or ulcers around the genital area

Chlamydia

This is the most serious, and the most common, curable sexually transmitted infection. It is the principal cause of infection of the uterus and Fallopian tubes. Chlamydia is also the main, and preventable, cause of pain during sexual intercourse, and the main cause of female infertility and ectopic pregnancy.

It is a particularly dangerous infection in that it is usually without symptoms and therefore frequently goes undetected. Nine out of ten chlamydial infections in women are acquired before the age of 25, and for women aged from

35 to 45, it is estimated that up to one-third may have been infected at some time in their lives.

Chlamydia is detected through cervical swab and an urethral sample. Treatment is by antibiotics.

Gonorrhoea

The long-term complications of gonorrhoea are usually less severe than those of chlamydia. Some two-thirds of men and one-third of women may notice symptoms. Diagnosis is made by swab and treatment is by antibiotics.

Syphilis

This infection has now reappeared in the West, following the epidemic in Eastern Europe and parts of Asia. It is transmitted during pregnancy and causes severe crippling disease to babies, but is completely curable with antibiotics. Antenatal screening is an essential part of prevention, both personally and nationally.

Herpes

The herpes simplex virus is present throughout the population. Some 60 per cent of people will be carrying it by their mid-twenties. Oral sex contributes to the spread of the virus.

Symptoms resemble those of flu, sometimes with headaches for about a week before the appearance of painful blisters. This is accompanied by tingling or numbness over a wider area of skin (the buttocks and the backs of the thighs), and sometimes by constipation and difficulty in passing urine. It is now established that herpes does not cause cervical cancer so annual smears are no longer required. Mother-to-baby transmission of herpes is very rare, but you can discuss with your obstetrician what procedure is necessary if herpes is present during labour.

When herpes occurs for the first time during pregnancy, it is nearly always the first visible attack rather than a newly acquired infection.

Hepatitis

The various hepatitis viruses can be transmitted in one of two ways: they are either passed from person to person in food and water (hepatitis A, E), or transmitted in blood and other infected body fluids through intimate contact (hepatitis B, D, C, and G).

Hepatitis is inflammation of the liver, which can occur either as a result of infection or through alcohol and drug abuse. However, the main causes of hepatitis are viruses.

The symptoms of all forms of viral hepatitis are similar. They range from a mild, flu-like syndrome to debility, nausea, vomiting, dark urine, light coloured stools, and yellowing of the skin and eyes. Hepatitis B and C can progress to chronic illness. In the most severe cases, coma and death can result. Some people with

35

acute or chronic hepatitis may experience no symptoms and the disease may pass unnoticed, yet they will still be infectious.

HIV

HIV infection now exists in over 140 countries, and over 8500 new HIV infections are diagnosed every day. There are only rarely signs or symptoms of HIV infection. People may be infected for years without realizing it, until the HIV develops into AIDS. Some people may experience a flu-like illness on first becoming infected and may then experience no further symptoms for many years.

HIV infection is transmitted from one person to another via the body fluids – blood, and seminal and vaginal fluids.

Anyone whose body fluids interchange with those of someone who is HIV positive risks becoming infected themselves. This can happen in any of these ways:

- sexual intercourse (both vaginal and anal)
- blood transfusion with infected blood
- use of needle or syringe that has already been used by someone with HIV infection
- babies can be infected through breast milk if the mother is HIV positive

HIV tests are available through your family doctor and through sexual health clinics. Further information can be obtained from national support and advice organizations (see pages 154–5).

Vaginal discharge

A vaginal discharge may occur for a number of reasons. It can be a symptom of sexually transmitted disease or of thrush (candida), which is not necessarily sexually transmitted. Any change in vaginal discharge should be investigated by your family doctor. Consult your doctor without delay if the discharge is yellowish and/or has a strong odour.

The hormonal changes that take place in early pregnancy can trigger thrush in up to one quarter of all women. Left untreated in pregnancy, thrush can be passed on to the newborn as neonatal oral thrush, which can make it difficult for babies to feed at this vital early stage.

Symptoms of thrush include vaginal discharge, unpleasant odour, sensation of itching, and swelling of the genital area. (See also PID on page 48.)

HOW TO PROTECT YOURSELF FROM STDS

- *Safe sex – always use a condom*
- *Avoid random sexual liaisons, as the consequences (such as infertility) may be serious*
- *Maintain good personal hygiene*
- *For women, seek immediate medical help if you suffer any persistent pelvic pain or discomfort other than your normal degree of menstrual discomfort*

36

The effects of alcohol

Men who are heavy drinkers may produce weak sperm that are unable to make the hazardous journey to meet the woman's egg. Male heavy drinkers can also produce babies with serious defects. Women who drink excessively, either around the time of conception or during pregnancy, can give birth to severely damaged babies.

Alcohol is a poison that damages the cells that make sperm. Prolonged heavy drinking may reduce the ability to make sperm in most men. Any delay in conception could be due to this.

While trying to conceive, it is advisable for a man to drink no more than two pints of beer or half a bottle of wine a day.

Many doctors maintain than an occasional drink will do no harm, while others advocate giving up alcohol altogether as part of pre-conceptual care and pregnancy. All doctors agree that heavy, regular drinking or binge drinking can adversely affect fertility and carries very high risks for the baby.

Two glasses of wine (not spirits) a week – at most – may do no harm to the pregnant woman, but alcohol crosses the placenta so the baby will be exposed to it. Spirits contain much more alcohol than wine or beer and should be avoided completely as part of pre-conceptual care and during the pregnancy itself.

If you have already had a child with a severe abnormality and are now trying for another baby, your partner should consider giving up drinking for three months before you attempt to conceive and continue to do so until you are sure that you are pregnant. You should refrain from drinking throughout your pregnancy.

Babies born to heavy drinkers may be affected by what is known as the fetal alcohol syndrome. This comprises a pattern of physical and mental defects including severe growth deficiency, heart defects, malformed facial features, a small head, abnormalities of co-ordination and movement, and mental impairment. Afflicted babies may be born addicted to alcohol and may suffer withdrawal symptoms, so that they seem twitchy and restless. They cannot feed properly and cannot thrive. They have to be sedated with drugs to help them through the withdrawal phase.

If you are at all concerned about your intake of alcohol and your ability to stop drinking at this crucial stage, speak to your doctor or consult the Finding help section of this book, pages 154–5.

Giving up smoking

It is well known that the single most important step anyone can take towards improving their health is to give up smoking. This is never more important than when becoming pregnant. Smoking reduces your fertility and is potentially harmful to your baby's health, to your own health, and to your partner's health.

Even if you were not to get enough sleep, never exercised, and did not eat particularly wisely, the fact that you continued to smoke in the first few months of your baby's life, while you are carrying her or him, is still the influence most likely to have a harmful effect on your child's health. Carbon monoxide and other poisonous chemicals from smoking cross the placenta and pass directly into the baby's bloodstream.

Women who smoke during pregnancy are more likely to miscarry or to have a stillbirth. If they carry the baby to term, the baby is likely to be underweight (usually referred to as low birth weight), and the child is more likely to suffer from infections of the respiratory tract. The child's memory and his or her ability to concentrate and learn may also be affected.

Babies of low birth weight are dysmature: although they are of the correct age to be delivered, they will not be as fully developed as a baby of normal weight and they will therefore be more vulnerable to infection and disease.

If you are already pregnant and still smoking, don't be tempted to think, "Well, it's too late now". It is not. You can minimize the damage by giving up now, or at least by cutting down drastically with the aim of giving up in two weeks' time.

Nicotine is a drug, which like many others is addictive, and it is undeniably difficult to kick the habit. However, if you give it up now, you will never have to go through the withdrawal symptoms again. Furthermore, you will be

THE EFFECTS OF SMOKING

Smoking causes the following in a healthy person:

rise in blood pressure • increase in pulse rate • irregular heartbeat • reduced efficiency of red blood cells responsible for carrying oxygen around the body; up to 15 per cent of them are subverted into carrying the carbon monoxide produced by smoke • decreased appetite • constipation • stimulation or depression of nervous system, depending on mood

doing your best to make sure that you give birth to a healthy and active child.

Tell yourself that not only are you storing up trouble for your child if you continue to smoke, but also for yourself.

Tobacco smoke contains dozens of carcinogens. It also contains carbon monoxide, a poisonous gas that lowers the amount of oxygen carried around the body by the blood. It does this by occupying the positions on red blood cells that are normally occupied by oxygen when it is carried around in the blood. Tobacco smoke also contains nicotine, which makes the heart beat faster and work harder than it should. Nicotine adversely affects blood-clotting factors, which may play a part in heart attacks. Tobacco smoke contains radioactive compounds, which are known to cause cancer, and hydrogen cyanide, which kills cilia, the tiny hairs that move together in waves to help keep our lungs clean and working efficiently.

When you smoke while you are pregnant, all these toxins enter your baby's bloodstream with every lungful you smoke. There could be no better time to give up smoking than before you try to conceive. If you need support, speak to your doctor or contact one of the organizations listed at the back of this book.

There is no better time for both you and your partner to kick the smoking habit than when you are trying to conceive. Giving up smoking for good will improve your own health and avoid harming your baby.

SMOKING-RELATED DISEASES

The chief diseases associated with regular smoking are:

cancer of the cervix • infertility • arteriosclerosis (hardening of the arteries) • atherosclerosis (narrowing of the arteries due to deposits of fat in their walls) • angina • heart attack • gangrene • stroke • bronchitis • cancer of the lung • emphysema • cancer of the oesophagus • cancer of the stomach • ulcer disease

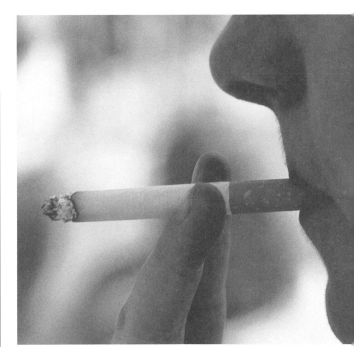

The wrong time

It is all-important to get the time of ovulation right when you are trying to conceive. Pregnancy cannot happen if sexual intercourse occurs too soon before ovulation and the sperm have died off before reaching the mature egg, or if sexual intercourse occurs too late and the sperm miss the egg.

Be sure that you know your fertile period (see pages 20–25). You can check your calculations with your family doctor if you are not sure. Note the first day of your periods for at least three months, preferably longer.

Lack of time

Some of us are too busy and simply forget to make love on exactly the right day. With a busy job and a good social life, it is very easy to let a few days go by – and they may be exactly the days on which you and your partner should have tried to conceive. You may be tired, your partner may be out – there could be many reasons. Be aware of your cycle and fertile period, and try to remember to make time for yourself and your partner to be together then.

Repeated miscarriage

Most miscarriages occur within the first two months of pregnancy, when many women are not yet aware of being pregnant. The loss of a

---

MISCARRIAGE: DANGER SIGNS

You should seek medical help without delay if you notice any of these symptoms at any stage of your pregnancy:

- *vaginal bleeding, unless it is merely spotting*
- *severe abdominal pain, especially if you are also bleeding vaginally*
- *cramps and backache similar to those of a period*
- *absence of the signs of pregnancy such as tender breasts and morning sickness*
- *continuous and severe headache, with or without blurred vision, and with or without swelling of the hands and ankles*
- *excessive vomiting in which you cannot keep down any food or liquid, even water*
- *breaking of the waters*
- *no fetal movements for 12 hours*

baby through miscarriage is much more common than many people believe.

Some leading gynaecologists estimate that the figure may be as high as 75 per cent of all pregnancies. Twenty years ago, it was believed that only 15 per cent of pregnancies were lost through miscarriage, but with improved screening and medical technology, it became

apparent that the figure was at least 20 per cent. In recent years the accepted figure has risen still higher, to 60 per cent.

After the first 12–16 weeks of pregnancy, miscarriage is much less likely to occur.

The definition of recurrent miscarriage is three miscarriages with no successful pregnancy in between. If you have experienced three miscarriages, you should seek professional advice.

There can be a number of warning signs for an impending miscarriage. Sadly, once a miscarriage starts, there is little that can be done to halt it.

MISCARRIAGE: CAUSES

The reasons for miscarriage are not yet fully understood but the known causes of miscarriage include:

- *mother contracts rubella, listeriosis, or chlamydia during pregnancy*
- *major abnormality of fetus or fertilized egg failing to implant in lining of uterus*
- *abnormality of the uterus, such as a large fibroid or polyps*
- *weak or incompetent cervix (a condition in which the cervix dilates instead of remaining tightly closed during pregnancy – this can be be corrected by a fairly straightforward procedure)*
- *certain antenatal tests carry a risk of miscarriage: these include chorionic villus sampling (1 in 100) and amniocentesis (1 in 200)*
- *mother has a pre-existing condition such as diabetes, epilepsy, asthma, kidney disease, or high blood pressure*

Grounds for investigation

Having one miscarriage, particularly in the early months of your pregnancy, does not mean that you are at greatly increased risk of another. However, there is no need simply to accept repeated miscarriages.

If you have had three miscarriages, you can be referred to a consultant gynaecologist for investigation. A late miscarriage – after 14 weeks – should also be investigated by a consultant gynaecologist.

Following investigation, you may then be referred on to a genetic counsellor, notably if there has been fetal abnormality, in order to determine the level of risk and discuss the best way forward. (See How genetics can help you, pages 56–61.)

41

Medical tests

Delayed conception is absolutely normal, and so infertility is defined as the inability to become pregnant after more than one year of regular, unprotected sexual intercourse.

What is the problem?

Some 15 to 20 per cent of couples have problems conceiving. In one third of cases, the problem lies with the woman having blocked Fallopian tubes; in one third again, the problem lies with the man's reproductive system (usually sperm abnormalities); and the remaining third comprises 20 per cent disorders of ovulation and 15 per cent unknown factors.

Tubal damage in the woman may have been caused by infection, miscarriage, ectopic pregnancy, or a number of other possibilities. This can sometimes be resolved surgically.

It must be said that even after investigation, some people remain infertile, although there is nothing apparently wrong with the reproductive system of either partner. Unexplained infertility can only be resolved through artificial insemination or assisted conception. This group also includes those for whom infertility may be caused by emotional factors: some people, for example, are unable to have sexual intercourse. If you feel your infertility may have an emotional cause, your doctor will be able to advise where to seek counselling.

Investigations

Once infertility is suspected, there are a number of medical procedures and investigations that can be carried out in order to establish the cause of the problem.

Blood hormone profiles

A blood test can be taken to see if the woman is ovulating. Blood progesterone levels can be measured in the second half of your menstrual cycle. Some clinics may measure the levels of hormones in the blood or urine every day for one menstrual cycle. Oestrogen, LH, progesterone, and prolactin may all be measured. If a woman has raised levels of the male hormone, testosterone, this may be the reason why she is not ovulating. This can be corrected with medication.

Semen analysis

Semen can be microscopically examined in a laboratory for volume, numbers of sperm, and sperm motility. It can also be examined for normality of sperm, infection, and the presence of antibodies that may be attacking the sperm.

42

Separation test

Commonly known as the swim test, despite the fact that sperm cannot actually swim, the separation test helps to determine the motility of the sperm.

Fructose measurement

If semen is low in fructose, which is produced by the seminal vesicles, it suggests that any blockage may be below the vesicles. This helps the surgeon locate and treat the blockage.

Testicular biopsy

Microscopic examination of a tissue sample shows whether the testis is producing sperm.

Human zona penetration test

For fertilization to occur, the sperm must be able to penetrate the zona or shell of the egg. To test this, the sperm are mixed with dead human eggs to see if they can penetrate them. In cases of infertility, none of the sperm may be strong enough to penetrate the zona or there may be so few that penetration is statistically unlikely.

Human zona attachment test

This involves counting the number of sperm that attach to the zona before penetrating it.

Testicular X-rays

X-rays of the testes help to determine the existence of any blockage and what treatment may be necessary.

Thermography

This is used to assess the temperature of the testicles. Some experts maintain that temperature is a defining factor in fertility, while others now disagree. This is a controversial issue, but this is the test used by those who believe it is important.

Karyotype (chromosome) test

This test determines whether or not there is a chromosomal problem with the sperm. Good sperm can be separated in the laboratory and artificial insemination used.

Skull X-ray and eye test

An X-ray of the skull along with an eye test enables the pituitary gland to be examined for LH or FSH production (see page 16). Irregular LH or FSH production can be treated with medication.

Thyroid hormone measurement

Thyroid problems are a rare cause of infertility but the thyroid should still be measured in any case. In case of problems it can be treated with medication.

Post-coital test

A sample of fluid is taken from the cervix within a few hours of sexual intercourse and examined to see if sperm are present and moving. This is a good test of the man's fertility and may also show that ovulation is occurring in the woman.

Sperm may be reaching the egg during the fertile period but may be unable to penetrate its outer wall. This is one of the causes of infertility that will be looked for in an investigation.

Crossed mucus penetration tests

If a post-coital test is repeatedly negative, the woman's mucus is combined with donor sperm, and the man's sperm with donor cervical mucus, in order to establish if it is the man or the woman who is producing antibodies that are killing off the sperm.

Endometrial biopsy

A microscopic examination of the lining of the uterus can determine whether or not progesterone is being produced.

Laparoscopy

This minor operation involves a small incision being made in the woman's abdomen. A special endoscope, the laparoscope, is passed through the abdomen allowing the uterus, Fallopian tubes, and ovaries to be viewed. Dye is passed through the neck of the uterus into the tubes to check for blockage or constriction. Abnormal growths or other problems will also be visible.

Hysteroscopy

This is similar to a laparoscopy but no incision is required. A specialized endoscope, the hysteroscope, is passed through the neck of the uterus to check for adhesions (scar tissue) and other problems.

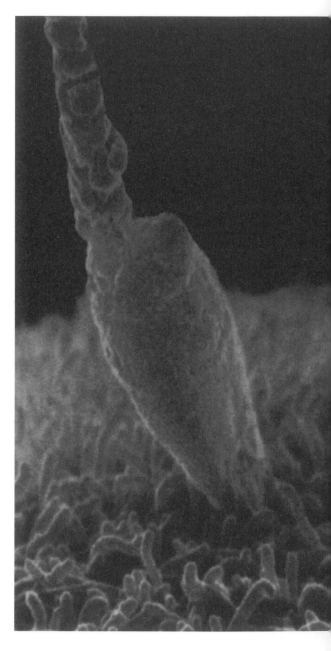

Hysterosalpinography

This X-ray technique employs a contrast (radio-opaque) medium injected into the uterus to outline the reproductive organs. This allows any blockage to be seen. This method is believed to identify 75 per cent of tubal blockages. It should be done early in the woman's menstrual cycle (within the first ten days) when she is least likely to be pregnant, as radiation can harm a developing fetus. This technique can cause some discomfort.

Hysterosalpingo-contrast sonography

This involves a contrast medium injected through the neck of the uterus. An ultrasound scan is performed, so that a probe can be introduced through the vagina. The contrast medium and ultrasound probe enable a detailed viewing of the women's reproductive system with minimal discomfort.

Following specialist investigations such as these, between 30 and 40 per cent of couples achieve a pregnancy within two years.

Possible problems

All the possible reasons for the inability to become pregnant are not yet fully understood, and the problem sometimes remains unexplained. However, some causes of infertility have been identified. They include the following:

Polycystic ovaries

Polycystic ovary syndrome is common and benign. It has no association with ovarian cancer or with the formation of large, medically significant cysts.

A polycystic ovary contains a collection of small fluid-filled cysts, which are each less than 5mm (¼in) in diameter. It affects about 1 in 10 women and the cause is unknown. However, some women who suffer from this condition will encounter a variety of hormonal problems, including infertility.

The typical features of polycystic ovary syndrome can include:

- obesity
- excessive hair growth on the face and/or body
- acne
- infrequent or no menstrual periods
- infertility

There is evidence to suggest that women with polycystic ovary syndrome may be more likely than unaffected women to develop diabetes mellitus and endometrial cancer.

Polycystic ovaries can be treated. There are a number of drug treatments now available that can induce ovulation and thus restore fertility. Procedures to treat the condition include the puncture and cauterization of the ovaries, using a needle during laparoscopy. In some women, this procedure alone can cause them to start ovulating regularly.

45

46

Early menopause

For most women, the menopause starts in their late forties and finishes with the final menstrual period in their early fifties. A premature menopause is when the last period occurs before the age of 40. This not uncommon condition affects one woman in every 100 and can affect women as young as 20 or even younger, who most probably will not even have started to think about getting pregnant and having children.

Women in their twenties and early thirties who experience premature menopause are more likely to suspect that their periods have stopped because of pregnancy rather than as a sign of menopause.

Symptoms of a premature menopause are caused by the fall in oestrogen levels that occurs as the ovaries stop producing eggs. The symptoms of premature menopause are therefore similar at whatever age the menopause occurs.

These symptoms include hot flushes, night sweats, insomnia, mood changes, anxiety, irritability, poor memory, poor concentration, loss of self-esteem, vaginal drying, painful intercourse, loss of libido, genito-urinary infections, thinning of the skin, splitting of the nails, aches and pains in the joints, and incontinence.

Laparoscopic investigation may show that the woman's ovaries no longer contain follicles with eggs. For those women who are unlucky enough to experience premature menopause, assisted conception is the only route to pregnancy and having a baby (see page 132).

Endometriosis

The endometrium is the lining of the uterus, which is shed during menstruation. Endometriosis is a condition in which cells similar to the type that normally line the inside of the uterus become established outside the uterus. This change can take place anywhere in the pelvic area – on either ovary, in either Fallopian tube, the bladder, the uterus, the bowel, the peritoneum, or on the pelvic wall.

Like those cells inside the uterus, these cells, called endometrial cells, respond to the changes in hormones that take place each month. During part of the month, they increase and, when the lining of the uterus is being shed in the form of a period, the endometriosis breaks down in the same way. However, because these cells are trapped inside the pelvic area, they cannot escape. Instead, they become inflamed and cause adhesions, which stick one internal organ to another.

As the cells spread, they can join organs to each other, or to the pelvic wall. These areas of tissue are called adhesions. They can form swellings which fill with dark blood, and these are known as chocolate cysts.

Endometriosis often goes undetected, with women attributing it simply to painful periods, yet it is a leading cause of infertility. One in ten women referred to gynaecologists has endometriosis, as it is a common condition.

Symptoms of endometriosis can include severe period pain, pain at the time of ovulation, during bowel movements, and during sexual intercourse, along with nausea and dizziness. Inability to become pregnant is a common symptom. It may be difficult to distinguish the symptoms of endometriosis from those of pelvic inflammatory disease.

Endometriosis is diagnosed by laparoscopic examination of the pelvis. This is a surgical procedure in which a tube with a tiny camera at one end is inserted into the pelvic area just below the navel.

The two main forms of treatment for endometriosis are:
• drug therapy with hormones
• surgery – endometriosis can be treated by laparoscopic surgery, using laser or cautery, or by laparotomy. In very severe cases, a hysterectomy may have to be considered.

A new form of treatment, the thermal coagulator, uses helium gas ionized by an electric current to dry out the endometriosis. It enables quick, safe, and accurate treatment.

After fertilization, the egg spends seven days travelling down the Fallopian tube. At this stage it develops into an embryo and is implanted in the endometrium: the lining of the uterus.

Endometriosis cannot be prevented but it is known that oral contraception and pregnancy help to protect against the condition.

Pelvic inflammatory disease

Pelvic inflammatory disease (PID) is an inflammation of the pelvic area, which includes the uterus, Fallopian tubes, and ovaries, due to infection.

PID is still not fully understood but it is now known to be due to a bacterial infection. Bacteria enter the body through the vagina and work their way up through the cervix into the pelvic cavity. The bacteria that are responsible for gonorrhoea and chlamydia (see pages 34–5) are thought to be the chief causes, although other bacteria, particularly some that normally exist harmlessly in the bowel or the gut, are also believed to play a part in PID.

PID can range from a mild condition with virtually no symptoms – other than an inability to become pregnant – to a very serious, occasionally life-threatening, disorder.

Symptoms include constant abdominal pain, which may become severe, or discomfort, weakness, fatigue, fever, and very heavy, painful periods. The pain usually manifests itself within a matter of hours and it feels like a dull ache across the lower abdomen. It may be so severe that the woman cannot move.

PID can cause infertility and it is estimated that women who have suffered with PID have a seven-fold risk of ectopic pregnancy. The scar tissue that is caused by PID can increase the risk of recurrent infection and cause pain during sex.

PID can occur as a consequence of chlamydia, childbirth, miscarriage, termination of pregnancy, and the fitting of an IUD (intrauterine device).

Diagnosis is usually made by internal examination and/or laparoscopy. PID is often not detected until investigations for delay or inability to become pregnant are carried out. It can often be mistaken for endometriosis and appendicitis. PID is usually treated with antibiotics, given in hospital intravenously or with oral antibiotics as an outpatient.

See also Sexual health check on pages 34–6.

Ectopic pregnancy

An ectopic pregnancy is a pregnancy that develops in the Fallopian tubes or occasionally elsewhere in the abdominal cavity rather than in the uterus. It is not known why this happens. It is known that an ectopic pregnancy is more likely if either of the Fallopian tubes has been damaged (by infection, by surgery, or by a previous ectopic pregnancy).

Ectopic pregnancy is a potentially serious condition, the symptoms of which can include very severe abdominal pain, vaginal spotting, and collapse. It can be mistaken initially for appendicitis or the threatened spontaneous miscarriage of a normal pregnancy.

Once an ectopic pregnancy is suspected or confirmed, an operation must be carried out to remove the pregnancy and, sometimes, part of the Fallopian tube and part of the ovary as well.

Women who have suffered one ectopic pregnancy are at greater risk of a subsequent one, and unfortunately the treatment for an ectopic pregnancy can cause tubal damage, leading to infertility. However, many women who have had an ectopic pregnancy go on to enjoy a normal pregnancy and delivery.

Polyps and fibroids

Polyps and fibroids are benign tumours or growths. It is not known why they develop. Polyps attach to a membrane by means of a stalk and they can occur either in the cervix or in the uterus. There may be no symptoms, although a cervical polyp may cause a watery discharge streaked with blood between periods and after intercourse.

Fibroids are benign tumours comprising bundles of muscle fibres that grow in the muscle wall of the uterus. They can vary in size from pea to football size. Fibroids are common, occurring in some 20 per cent of women over 30, often without producing any symptoms.

Symptoms that may occur include heavy menstrual bleeding, including flooding, passing clots of blood, and long-lasting periods.

Associated anaemia can produce feelings of exhaustion, breathlessness, and depression. Other symptoms include severe cramps, incontinence, dribbling, constipation, cystitis, and inability to become pregnant.

Diagnosis is by internal examination, ultrasound scan, hysteroscopy, laparoscopy, or hysterosalpingogram. Treatment options available include TCRE (transcervical resection of the endometrium), medication, and surgery. The two operations available are myomectomy (removal of fibroids, leaving uterus intact), and hysterectomy (either full or partial).

DANGER SIGNS FOR AN ECTOPIC PREGNANCY

- *sudden, sharp, or persistent pain in lower abdomen*
- *pain that feels as though it is under one of the shoulder blades*
- *vaginal spotting*

HELP IS AT HAND

It is reassuring to know that 30–40 per cent of couples achieve a pregnancy within two years following specialist investigation. For those couples who are still unable to conceive, a number of options remain available, as explored on pages 118–41.

49

Planning
your pregnancy

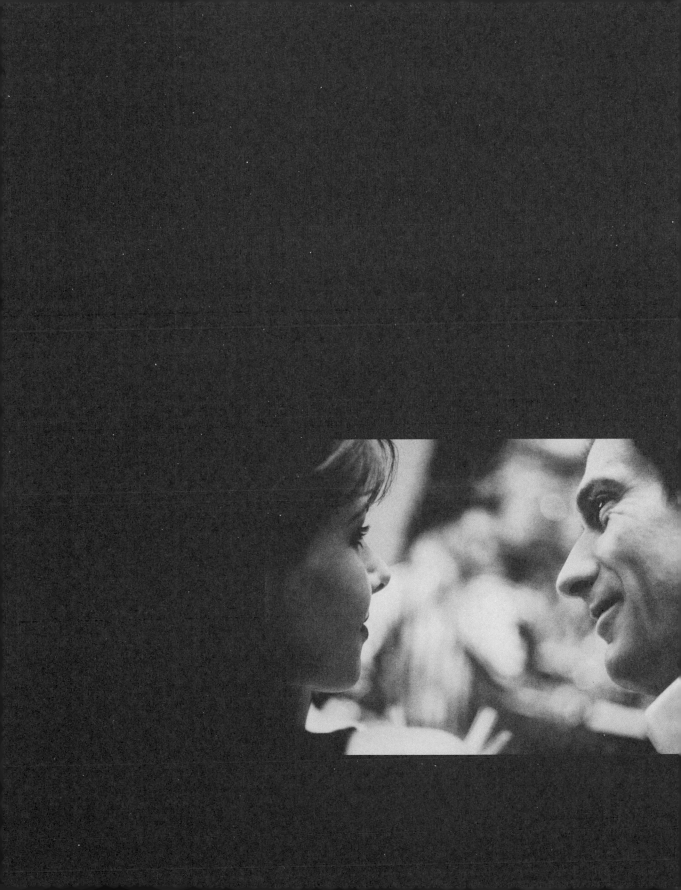

Health check-ups and immunization

Your individual and family medical histories are significant in pre-pregnancy planning. Your own medical history, including menstrual problems, infections, STDs, pre-existing health problems, rubella immunity (see page 56), and dental care, all need to be taken into account as part of your pre-conceptual care.

If you or any of your family have any condition that is a potential risk factor for pregnancy, you may wish to see a genetic counsellor (through your family doctor), in order to discuss the best way forward (see pages 56–61).

Risk factors for pregnancy
- age less than 18
- age 36 and over
- 4 or more previous deliveries
- IUD in place
- previous stillbirth or neonatal death
- previous small baby or previous large baby
- previous Caesarean, hysterotomy, or myomectomy
- two or more miscarriages before existing pregnancy
- in a previous pregnancy, early labour, cervical stitch, late miscarriage or termination, two or more terminations
- congenital fetal abnormality in previous baby
- antibodies in previous pregnancy that could harm the fetus, such as rhesus antibodies
- in previous pregnancies, pre-eclampsia, hypertension, and proteinuria
- severe bleeding after giving birth or manual removal of placenta
- very short labour (less than 2 hours) or long labour (over 12 hours)
- postnatal depression after birth of previous baby
- uterine problem such as fibroids
- blood disorder
- family history of diabetes or congenital fetal abnormality
- smoking
- drinking more than ten units of alcohol a week
- drug misuse by either parent

PREGNANCY SCREENING

Blood tests check for the following:

- *your blood group and whether you are rhesus positive or rhesus negative (see page 56)*
- *anaemia*
- *immunity to rubella*
- *blood sugar level (not routine in some units)*
- *hepatitis B*
- *HIV, if you are in a high-risk group or if you ask for the test*
- *syphilis (chlamydia and gonorrhoea may also be checked for routinely)*

A urine test checks for kidney disease, diabetes, and urinary tract disease such as cystitis. You will also need to have a cervical smear and an ultrasound scan.

- several different sexual partners, anal intercourse, bisexual partner
- hepatitis B, HIV, AIDS
- high blood pressure (140/90 or more, after you have been lying down for 5 minutes)
- underweight or overweight (a BMI of less than 20 or more than 30)
- less than 1.52m (5ft) tall
- protein in urine
- heart murmur
- pelvic or abdominal abnormalities
- unexpected vaginal bleeding

If you are of Afro-Caribbean origin, a test for sickle-cell disease is usually recommended. Similarly, if you are of Mediterranean or Asian origin, a test for thalassemia is advised.

Such a long list can look very daunting, but it helps the hospital team to identify any risks in your pregnancy so that they can offer you the appropriate tests, and ensure that you are fully prepared for any complications.

How to tell if you are pregnant

Some women know very quickly that they are pregnant, but most need something more than a missed period. Pregnancy can be confirmed by a positive pregnancy test result or an ultrasound scan. If you are not overweight, a scan through the abdominal wall can see the baby's heartbeat after seven weeks. Before that, a trans-vaginal scan will show the fetal heart.

Common early signs include feeling sick, feeling tired, needing to pass water more often than usual, swollen and tender breasts, constipation, disliking foods that you normally relish, and craving foods that you don't usually want, and a significant absence of the irritability and other symptoms associated with PMT.

You can obtain a pregnancy test at your doctor's surgery, at a family planning clinic, or you can buy one from a pharmacy, though over-the-counter test kits are not fully reliable. Pregnancy testing can be carried out within days of a missed period.

53

Improving your chances of conception

All the elements that will help you conceive need to be integrated into your and your partner's lifestyle, without letting your desire to have a baby overshadow the other things that are important to you in your life together.

Helping yourself

The best chances of conceiving a baby, as we saw earlier, can be summarized as follows:

- Calculating your fertile period
- If you are taking the contraceptive pill, some doctors will recommend that you change to a barrier method of contraception for a few months so that your periods are re-established before you attempt to conceive. However, some specialists regard this change as unnecessary
- Making love frequently (say, every 24 hours) during the fertile period
- Both partners cutting down on alcohol
- Both partners giving up smoking
- Following a good, healthy diet (see pages 62–117)
- Achieving a healthy Body Mass Index (see page 32) through a combination of exercise and good food
- Getting sufficient good quality sleep

- Remembering to drink eight glasses of water every day
- Taking 0.4mg folic acid as a daily supplement in order to prevent neural tube defect (which affects 1–2 in every 1000 babies). There is evidence that folic acid (a B vitamin) may be beneficial in reducing the chances of having a baby with spina bifida and other neural tube defects.
- Resolving any medical problems that either you or your partner is aware of through your family doctor
- Resolving any other problems that may be causing either you or your partner stress
- And finally – just as important as everything else in the list – giving each other treats (see pages 92–117).

Anxiety and emotional factors can be a significant and substantial cause of delay in getting pregnant and a sense of perspective is, therefore, all-important.

54

YOUR STRESS RATING

The most commonly used and well-established rating for stress is that composed by Holmes and Rahe in 1967. This enables you to assess the stresses in your life over the past 12 months. Out of the following list, tick all the events that you have experienced in the last year:

death of spouse	100	*son or daughter leaving home*	29
divorce	73	*trouble with in-laws*	29
marital separation	65	*outstanding personal achievement*	28
prison term	63	*spouse begins or stops work*	26
death of a close family member	63	*starting or finishing school*	26
personal injury or illness	53	*change in living conditions*	25
marriage	50	*change of personal habits*	24
loss of job	47	*trouble with boss*	23
marital reconciliation	45	*change in work hours or conditions*	20
retirement	45	*change in residence*	20
change in family member's health	44	*change in school*	20
pregnancy	40	*change in recreational habits*	19
sex difficulties	39	*change in church activities*	19
addition to family	39	*change in social activities*	18
business readjustment	39	*taking out a small mortgage/loan*	17
change in financial state	38	*change in sleeping habits*	16
death of a close friend	37	*more/fewer family gatherings*	15
change to different type of work	36	*change in eating habits*	15
more/fewer marital arguments	35	*holiday*	13
taking out a large mortgage or loan	31	*Christmas*	12
foreclosure on mortgage or loan	30	*minor violation of the law*	11
change in work responsibilities	29		

Assess your stress rating by adding the figures for each life event.

If your total comes to less than 150, you have no more than the average risk of illness (30 per cent). If your total comes to between 150 and 299, you have a 50 per cent probability of developing an illness as a direct consequence of your stress levels. Put simply, the higher your score, the higher your stress levels, and the greater the possible risk this level of stress may have on your fertility.

How genetics can help you

The study of genetics and the introduction of genetic counselling have already proved invaluable to many prospective parents who may have risk factors in their personal medical history or family medical history that could affect a pregnancy and the birth of a healthy child.

Genetic counselling may be offered to women who are over 35 to evaluate the risk factor of age. Counselling will also be offered to those who have experienced repeated (more than three) miscarriages.

Before we look at the relatively rare genetic and chromosomal disorders, we should consider the potential complications of rubella and rhesus, both of which are relatively common, both of which can be screened for before you attempt to conceive, and both of which will be screened for, in any case, as part of your antenatal care.

Rubella

If you develop rubella (formerly known as German measles) during pregnancy, and particularly during the first three months (when you may not even know you are pregnant), the baby may be severely affected. The virus can attack the baby's nervous system and heart and can cause deformity, deafness, blindness, miscarriage, or stillbirth.

Rubella is highly infectious, particularly at the time that any rash appears. However, it is also infectious for a week before and a week after any rash. The incubation period is between 14 and 21 days.

Rubella can exist in a very mild form and can be mistaken for a cold. Ideally, you should be checked to establish your immunity to rubella before you attempt to become pregnant. If you are not immune, you can be vaccinated and then be checked again to ensure that the vaccine has worked.

It is important to have the rubella immunity test, even if you are certain that you had rubella as a child, because rubella is a virus that is often misdiagnosed, and it is uncertain for how long immunity achieved in this way lasts.

Rhesus factor

Most people are rhesus positive but some 15 per cent (1 in 6) are rhesus negative. Rhesus positive blood cells possess an antigen that can stimulate the production of antibodies to fight alien blood cells. Rhesus negative blood lacks this antigen. A problem arises in pregnancy only if you are rhesus negative (R-).

If you are R-, and the baby has the same blood group as you, but is rhesus positive (R+), some of the blood cells that escape from its body into yours during pregnancy, and especially during the birth, will provoke your body into making antibodies to fight the alien cells and destroy them.

This does not usually harm either you or the baby. The problem of the rhesus factor only arises with second and subsequent pregnancies, if the fetus is again R+ and the mother, of course, is still R-.

Following the first pregnancy, the woman's body will now contain antibodies to fight and destroy rhesus positive cells. These antibodies can pass into the circulation of the second baby, where they will break down its cells. This can lead to stillbirth, or a baby with severe anaemia, heart failure, extreme jaundice, spasticity, or mental impairment.

A woman with rhesus negative blood, who has developed antibodies as a consequence of a previous pregnancy, will therefore need special care to ensure that the antibodies in her blood are not able to destroy the blood cells of her growing baby.

Any rhesus negative woman who has any invasive procedure, such as chorionic villus sampling, cordocentesis, and amniocentesis, must be given anti-D gamma globulin injections on these occasions. The injections are given after the test procedure in order to prevent the problems that would be caused by leakage of the baby's blood cells into her bloodstream. They are also given after the birth of her first child and subsequent children in order to destroy the antibodies.

If the woman does develop antibodies and these are identified during pregnancy, the baby may be transfused (given a blood transfusion), while it is still in the uterus.

Screening for rare disorders

If your personal medical history, or that of your partner, or either of your families' histories suggests a risk of a rare disorder, you can have genetic counselling and testing in order to assess the degree of risk.

Genetics is the science of heredity. The overall incidence of single-gene disorders is at least 1 in 100 live births and that of chromosomal abnormalities is at least 1 in 150 at birth. About 25 per cent of all children occupying a hospital bed are there because of a genetic problem.

Genetic counselling is the process by which patients or relatives at risk of suffering from, or passing on, a hereditary disorder are advised of the consequences of that disorder. The presence of some of these diseases can be tested for, pre-conceptually, by means of a simple blood test.

Single-gene diseases

It is thought that around 4000 diseases are caused by a mutation in a single gene that is inherited from one or both parents. However, most of these disorders are very rare, accounting for only about 3 per cent of all disease.

> ### SOME OF THE MOST COMMON INHERITED DISORDERS:
>
> - *Congenital heart defects (encompasses a variety of malformations)*
> - *Familial adenomatous polyposis (colon cancer)*
> - *Polycystic kidney disease*
> - *Hemochromatosis (iron storage disease)*
> - *Neural tube defects (defects of the spinal cord)*
> - *Hypercholesterolemia*
> - *Diabetes, type 1*
> - *Breast and ovarian cancer*
> - *Cleft lip and palate*
> - *Down's Syndrome*
> - *Fragile X syndrome (leading cause of mental impairment)*
> - *Sickle-cell anaemia*
> - *Cystic fibrosis*
> - *Duchenne Muscular Dystrophy*
> - *Haemophilia A*
> - *Marfan Syndrome*

Some diseases occur more frequently in certain ethnic groups. Among the more common inherited disorders for which single, causative genes have been identified are sickle-cell anaemia (Afro-Caribbeans, African Americans, and Hispanics), cystic fibrosis (Caucasians), and Tay-Sachs (Ashkenazi Jews).

Mutations

While most DNA variation is normal, harmful sequence changes sometimes occur in our DNA that cause or contribute to disease. All DNA sequence changes – called mutations – are either passed down from parent to child (in the sperm or egg cells), or acquired during a person's lifetime.

Most diseases are due to acquired changes, known as sporadic mutations. These mutations can arise spontaneously during normal functions, as when a cell divides, or in response to environmental stresses such as toxins, radiation, hormones, and perhaps even diet.

Nature provides us with a system of finely tuned repair enzymes that find and fix most DNA errors. However, as we age, our repair systems may become less efficient and allow us to accumulate uncorrected mutations. This can result in diseases such as cancer.

Depending on where in our genome they occur, mutations can have devastating effects or none at all. If they are small and fall in the vast areas of non-coding sequences, no one

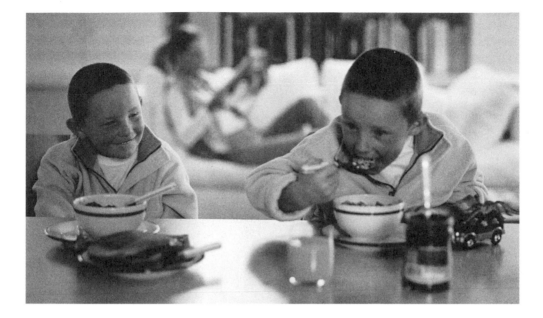

might be any the wiser. Changes within genes, however, can result in faulty proteins that function at less than normal levels or those that are completely non-functional, causing disease.

Sometimes, only a tiny change in a DNA sequence will lead to a serious disease. The substitution of just a single base (see page 60), for example, leads to sickle-cell anaemia. Other diseases are caused by deletions or additions of single or multiple bases. Too many repetitions of a particular sequence of three DNA bases can cause Huntington's disease, a fatal neurological disorder; Fragile X syndrome, the most common form of inherited mental impairment; or myotonic dystrophy, a muscle-

Identical twins are born when a single fertilized egg divides completely and equally at a very early stage of embryonic development. The two children therefore share the same genetic blueprint.

wasting disease. Other diseases can result from large rearrangements of DNA.

For most diseases, the causes are much more complex than just gene mutations. The common disorders are thought to be due to a variety of gene mutations, perhaps acting together, or to a combination of gene mutations and environmental factors. Heart disease, diabetes, hypertension, cancers, Alzheimer's disease (AD), schizophrenia, and manic depression are all examples of complex diseases.

What are genes?

A gene is simply a piece of DNA, the chemical responsible for storing and transferring all hereditary information in a cell. Genes accomplish this by containing recipes for making proteins, the workhorses of all our trillions of cells. All living organisms are made up largely of proteins, which provide the structural components of all our cells and tissues, as well as specialized enzymes for all essential chemical reactions.

Through these proteins, our genes determine how well we process foods, detoxify poisons, and respond to infections. Although our cells have the same genes, not all genes are active in all cells. Heart cells synthesize proteins required for that organ's structure and function, liver cells make liver proteins, and so on.

In humans and other higher organisms, a DNA molecule consists of two ribbon-like strands that wrap around each other, resembling a twisted ladder. The ladder rungs are made up of chemicals called bases, with the abbreviations A, T, C, and G. Each rung consists of a pair of bases, either A and T, or C and G. We have three billion base pairs (six billion bases) of DNA in most of our cells: this is our genome.

With the exception of identical twins, the sequence of the bases – the order of As, Ts, Cs, and Gs – is different for every one of us, which is what makes each of us unique. Variation in the base sequence, along with environmental factors, accounts for all our human diversity, including disease.

Every human being has between 30,000 and 40,000 genes, according to research published in February 2001, which is far fewer than was originally believed. These genes determine hair colour and eye colour, type of build, and other traits. The genes are like tiny switches that direct the growth and development of every part of our physical and biochemical systems. Genes are packed into each of the chromosomes inside most of our cells.

Sperm and egg cells are different from other body cells. These reproductive cells each have only 23 unpaired chromosomes. When a single sperm and egg come together, forming their own new cell with 46 chromosomes, pregnancy begins. Thus the baby is genetically unique, with a genetic blueprint half of which comes from the mother and half from the father.

The chromosomes

The DNA making up our genome is divided into tightly coiled packets called chromosomes, which reside in the nucleus of each cell. Each chromosome is a single DNA molecule, and lengths vary from 50 million to 250 million bases. Scientists can distinguish the chromosomes by size, distinctive staining patterns, and other characteristics.

Most cells have 46 chromosomes, 23 from each parent. A set of 23 contains 22 numbered chromosomes (1–22) plus either an X or Y sex-determining chromosome. Females get an X from each parent, and males get an X and a Y.

Chromosomes are not continuous strings of genes. The genes are interspersed among millions of bases of DNA that do not code for proteins (non-coding DNA), and whose functions are largely unknown. In fact, genes constitute only part of the human genome.

Different types of defects

The four different types of genetic disorder are:

- Single-gene defects (responsible for about 4000 diseases)
- Dominant genetic disease (such as hypercholesterolaemia and Huntington's chorea)
- Recessive genetic disease (such as cystic fibrosis, carried by 1 in 20 of the population, and thalassemia, which is common in certain ethnic groups)
- Sex-linked disorders (these are usually passed on by the female but only boys are affected)

There are also:

- Chromosomal defects (in which one or more chromosomes carrying many genes are abnormal)
- Congenital malformations (such as spina bifida, a neural tube defect)
- Illnesses with a genetic component

Assessing test results

No genetic test will produce a result that declares an absolute Yes or No. Test results show only a likelihood – an estimated risk – of developing a particular inherited disease, or of conceiving a child who may develop the disease. The estimated risk has to be evaluated by a genetic counsellor who takes all other factors into account.

This estimated risk is then discussed by both partners with the genetic counsellor. Other medical specialists may also possibly be consulted, so that the couple may decide the best way forward. (See also Knowing when to seek help, pages 132–41, and Finding help, pages 154–5.)

Some in vitro fertilization (IVF) clinics can offer prospective parents who are at high risk from some genetic diseases a way to ensure that they will not pass on the defective gene to their children. The clinics also offer parents the option of remaining ignorant of their own genetic status, which many prefer.

After fertilization of the egg outside the mother's body, the resulting embryos are tested for gene mutations associated with a particular disease, and embryos without the mutation are selected for implantation in the uterus.

61

Eating well and staying in shape

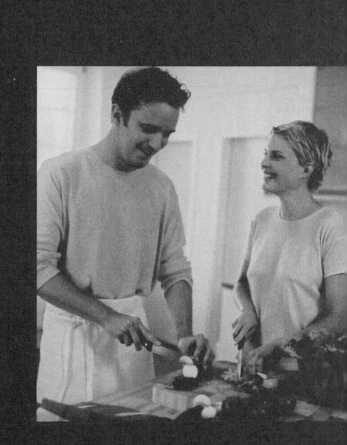

Lifestyle choices

Eating well and staying fit is as much about your lifestyle – how you live – as what you eat and how much you exercise. It is important to be aware of the right ingredients for a healthy life, to try to incorporate some of them into your way of life, and to maintain a sensible balance between your working day and your home life with your family and friends.

This chapter offers, as well as guidelines for eating healthily and well, a number of techniques for staying fit through exercise and a range of the available complementary techniques. The ideal is to eat well, exercise regularly, and incorporate, if you wish, a couple of the complementary therapies of your choice.

Exercise and complementary therapies are particularly valuable in alleviating stress and tension. Exercise in the fresh air, such as walking and cycling, is especially healthy and tones up all the muscles of the body.

It is important to strengthen your immune system through regular, healthy eating before attempting to conceive in order to ward off any ailments such as colds and flu that could occur during your subsequent pregnancy. You should bear in mind that many drugs, even those that alleviate common ailments, cannot be taken during pregnancy.

A lifestyle that incorporates the twin ingredients of eating well and staying fit will stand you and your whole family in good stead

for many years to come. It is important for babies and young children to become accustomed in their early years to healthy eating and to regular exercise. The combination of the two is much more useful to good health than either diet or exercise alone.

The habits that you put in place now, while you are attempting to conceive, should become the foundation of your family lifestyle in the future. Healthy practices should be ingrained into your lifestyle, so that they become automatic, and not something that you have to make an effort to be concerned with.

Your BMI, or Body Mass Index (see page 32), provides a quick method of assessing whether you are eating not only healthily but also the correct amount.

How much to eat

A baby's health is entirely dependent on what the woman eats and drinks just before and during pregnancy. It used to be believed that

64

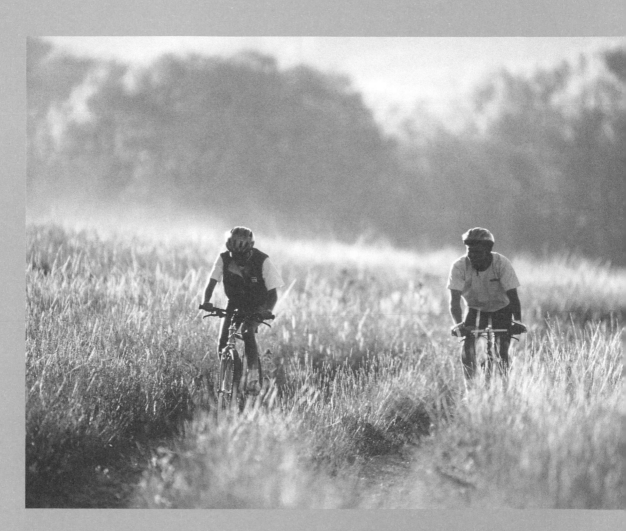

the mother should "eat for two" but this is no longer regarded as sensible. Some medical advice even went too far in the other direction and suggested that pregnant women should deliberately avoid "eating for two". This led many pregnant women to eat inadequate amounts of food, so afraid were they of gaining

Good exercise need not – indeed should not – mean boring hours pounding away on a treadmill in the gym. Find an activity that gives you pleasure, preferably in the open air. Cycling, fast walking and swimming are all excellent aerobic exercises that will tone all the muscles in your body, as well as your cardiovascular system. They are also enjoyable and sociable, and allow you to become fit and healthy, while spending time with your partner.

weight. Needless to say, this anxiety led to some pregnancies that were fraught with problems, resulting in difficult labours and underweight, poorly babies.

Weight gain in pregnancy

Women who gain a reasonable amount of weight, on the other hand, tend to have easier pregnancies and labours, with a lower incidence of miscarriage and neonatal deaths (deaths at around the time of delivery). Heavier babies usually tend to be healthier, and they are also, as a rule, better able to resist common childhood ailments and infections.

Having said this, mothers who gain far too much weight during pregnancy can develop diabetes. Their babies then run a higher risk of developing diabetes themselves.

Fertility depends on a great many factors, with good diet being only one of them. However, diet does have a profound effect on fertility. For example, there is evidence to suggest that the number of births in a population declines during times of food shortage.

A pregnant woman needs to lay down fat early in her pregnancy in preparation for producing milk and breastfeeding. These stores of fat will remain after delivery but will usually gradually disappear with breastfeeding and regular exercise.

Not all the weight gain is made up of fat. The placenta, the fluids surrounding the baby, and the baby itself, account for over half the total weight gain. During pregnancy, the volume of blood manufactured by a woman's body is increased by about 1.5 litres (2.5 pints). This extra blood, which also contributes to the total weight gain, is needed by the uterus, the breasts, and the other vital organs to sustain and support a healthy pregnancy.

Most women gain between 9 and 13.5kg (20–30lb) during pregnancy. The amount of and rate of weight gain varies from individual to individual, thus making it wrong to lay down any hard and fast rules about how much weight you should or should not put on. It is obvious, though, that no pregnant woman should be on a weight-reducing diet.

The woman who is already overweight before her pregnancy may not need to gain as much weight during pregnancy as the woman who is underweight, but she should certainly not be thinking about slimming once she knows that

RATE OF WEIGHT GAIN

A woman's weight may be monitored once she knows she is pregnant. The amount each woman gains will vary, but the rate of gain is likely to be approximately as follows:

0–12 weeks	*10 per cent*
13–20 weeks	*25 per cent*
21–28 weeks	*45 per cent*
29–36 weeks	*20 per cent*
37–40 weeks	*0 per cent*

66

she is pregnant. You are less likely to gain weight once you know that you are pregnant if you follow the traditional, sound advice: breakfast like a king, lunch like a prince, and dine like a pauper. In other words, make sure that you eat a healthy and sustaining breakfast, a good lunch, and a small, nutritious low-fat dinner (see page 69).

Minimal contact

When you are attempting to conceive a baby, or if you are already pregnant, you should avoid contact with the following as far as possible:

X-rays – have any medical investigation, if possible, and any dental work, carried out before you attempt to conceive.

Mobile phones – as the research evidence concerning the effect on the brain and the nervous system is not yet clear, reduce your use to a minimum.

Cats and kittens – their faeces may lead to the pregnant woman contracting an infectious condition called toxoplasmosis, which can harm a developing fetus and cause a variety of abnormalities. The principal hazard is through having contact with the faeces of kittens in the first year of their life. Kittens' faeces are infectious only when the kittens first acquire toxoplasmosis. They develop antibodies to the infection and excrete the parasite. Kittens or young cats acquire the infection through hunting and it is statistically likely that they will become infected in the first year of life. Thereafter, they will not be infectious. Never empty cat litter trays unless you are wearing gloves; and disinfect cat litter trays with boiling water for 5 minutes every day.

Garden soil may contain the agent that leads to toxoplasmosis. Always wear gloves for gardening and wash your hands after any contact with soil. (See also pages 76–7.)

Steak tartare and any other forms of raw and very rare beef, or other forms of meat, irrespective of country of origin, should be avoided due to risk of BSE and toxoplasmosis.

Long-haul flights are known to carry a risk of DVT (deep vein thrombosis). Leave your seat every hour and move around. In between times, flex your wrists and ankles and stretch your neck to left, to right, and downwards in order to keep freshly oxygenated blood flowing around your body. Drink plenty of water and avoid alcohol.

Televisions and computers give out small amounts of radiation but, we are told, not in sufficient quantity or strength to have an effect on fertility or pregnancy, provided that your use is not excessive.

67

Your diet

Eating well and regularly is of paramount importance for you and your partner when you are trying to conceive a baby.

Is your food safe?

Pregnant women and women who hope to become pregnant are at particular risk of food poisoning, which can manifest itself in a number of unpleasant and potentially damaging ways, such as listeria, E. coli, salmonella, and Campylobacter pylori. Other groups at risk of food poisoning are babies and children under the age of seven, people over the age of 65, and anyone who is already ill or who has any kind of immune system deficiency or disorder.

As many as 1 in 5 people can expect an episode of diarrhoea and vomiting every year. The chief offender is known to be campylobacter, which far outweighs the other causes such as salmonella and E. coli.

How you eat
How you prepare food

The less that food is cooked, the better it is for your body and your immune system. It's a good idea to eat as much raw food – such as salads and fruit – as you can. Conversely, the more highly processed food is, the less likely it is to

THE SEVEN ESSENTIALS OF FOOD HYGIENE

- *Wash your hands in hot water with an antibacterial preparation before and after handling any food (including poultry, raw meat, fish, seafood, salads, vegetables, and eggs).*

- *Wash your hands in hot water with an antibacterial preparation after handling domestic pets and, particularly, cat litter and kitten litter (because of the risk of toxoplasmosis, see page 67).*

- *Kitchen surfaces should be disinfected with an antibacterial solution.*

- *Wooden chopping boards (which trap bacteria) should be replaced with plastic ones, which should be disinfected after each use.*

- *Raw foods should be stored separately from cooked foods. Always follow the Use By date.*

- *Refrigerators should be maintained at under 5°C. Use a thermometer.*

- *All taps and telephones should be washed with an antibacterial solution. (How often do you stop preparing food to answer the phone?)*

be nutritious, and the more likely it is to contain toxins that will be harmful to you.

In the mornings, go for wholemeal bread, muesli, yoghurt, and fruit. Salads, uncooked vegetables, wholemeal pastas, and white fish are all excellent for lunch or supper. Most vegetables are much tastier and much more potent system cleansers and detoxifiers when eaten uncooked. Choose from carrot, baby corn, broccoli, white cabbage, tomato, celery, mangetout, mushroom, courgette, finely chopped onion, shallot, and leek.

When you eat

Stoking up the fire of your metabolism in the morning is a must for a healthy reproductive system. Making your body run on empty for half the day puts a stress on it, so always find time for breakfast.

How often you eat

It is much easier for the brain and body to function if they are nourished at regular, short intervals. It is preferable to have six tiny meals a day rather than a couple of large ones, even though this may not always be practicable. Never miss a meal as this allows toxins to build up in your body and your system slows down.

Water of life

Water is essential for a healthy functioning body. Fatigue is one of the early warning signs of dehydration, which makes the body more

TIPS FOR HEALTHY EATING

Never eat in a hurry • Don't eat more than you need • Always drink water with a meal • Never skip breakfast • Never embark on a faddy or gimmicky diet • Don't go for meal replacements in any form • Don't miss meals • Ignore cravings and give up junk foods and highly processed foods • Cut down on alcohol • Don't go supermarket shopping when you are hungry – eat first • Four, five, or six small meals a day are much better for your body than two or three larger meals a day • Eat slowly and don't try to do something else while you are eating: that way your digestive system is more likely to work efficiently • Never resort to packaged and convenience foods

69

vulnerable to infections and viruses, and generally weakens all the systems of the body.

Drink eight long glasses of water throughout the day to feel invigorated: first thing in the morning, mid-morning, before lunch, after lunch, mid-afternoon, before supper, after supper, and shortly before going to bed.

What you eat

In order to maintain a healthy balanced diet, you need to eat from the following food groups every day. You should also eat five helpings of vegetables every day for optimum health.

Meat, poultry, and fish provide protein. Beef, lamb, pork, and bacon are all good sources of protein. Go for lean cuts and trim off any visible fat before cooking. Grill, roast, or microwave meat, so that some of the fat drains off. If you are making a casserole or stew, add more vegetables than meat so that you have a healthier balance of foods.

Fish and poultry are better for you than red meat. Fish is a great source of protein and is low in saturates. Mackerel, tuna, salmon, and sardines are rich in fish oils, which offer good health benefits. Grill, microwave, steam, or bake your fish rather than deep frying, in order to avoid eating saturates.

Dairy products supply smaller amounts of protein and calcium from foods such as eggs, cheese, milk, and milk products.

Women who wish to become pregnant or are already pregnant, should avoid raw or lightly cooked eggs or egg whites (found in foods such as softly cooked omelettes, home-made mayonnaise, mousse, or as a binding for hamburgers) because of the risk of salmonella. They should also avoid eating soft cheeses such as Brie and Camembert because of the risk of listeria.

If you are worried about weight gain, reduce your butter intake. Yoghurt is a good alternative to cream. Natural yoghurt is the healthy option. Try adding chopped fresh fruit or whizzing the fruit and the yoghurt in the blender to make a healthy pudding or drink.

Nuts, peas, lentils, soya, and pulses provide protein. Peas and beans, as well as other vegetables, also provide essential vitamins, as well as being a good source of fibre. Fibre is an indigestible substance obtained from nuts, cereals, fruit, and vegetables. It is not broken down or digested in the body, but it is essential to health because it speeds up the passage of waste products through the bowel and helps to remove toxins from the body. Fibre aids the digestive processes, and so helps to keep all systems of the body functioning well.

Carbohydrate and fibre are supplied by pulses and grains in the form of wholewheat cereal, wholemeal bread, wholemeal pasta, and wholemeal savoury biscuits such as oatcakes. Smaller amounts of fibre can also be derived from vegetables.

Go for wholewheat breakfast cereals or, preferably, muesli. Avoid any brands with added sugar and honey. In the case of noodles and pasta, choose wholewheat pasta, which is bulkier, much higher in fibre, and less fattening than processed white pasta. It also has a delicious nutty taste, which is complemented by tomato and vegetable-based sauces. If you are watching your weight, increase the amount of wholewheat pasta you eat and keep the sauce to a minimum. When choosing rice, go for brown rice or wild rice. Again, these have a nutty flavour and blend deliciously with robust vegetable sauces.

Provided that you eat at regular times and choose foods from the groups described, you will be following a nutritious and healthy diet. You should not need any added vitamins or minerals, either before or during pregnancy, other than folic acid (see list on page 73).

The importance of fibre

Fibre is especially important, both pre-conceptually and during pregnancy, because of its role in relieving constipation, which leads to feelings of fatigue and general sluggishness.

Pre-conceptually, a high fibre content is an essential element of a healthy diet, helping the body's digestive system to eliminate waste products and toxins – which would otherwise be accumulated in the body – as quickly as possible. Fibre acts as an indigestible bulking agent, helping to propel other foods through the gastrointestinal tract with the minimum of delay and thus assisting in regular evacuation of the bowel. Fibre is just as important when you are expecting your baby, as constipation is a common complaint of pregnancy.

Constipation is apt to occur during pregnancy because of the effect of the pregnancy hormones, which slow down bowel movements. Constipation is very often a sign of insufficient fibre in the diet and of not drinking enough water.

A fibre-rich diet would include muesli and wholewheat bread for breakfast, wholewheat pasta or bread with plenty of vegetables and fruit at lunchtime, and more vegetables, vegetable-based dishes, or salads, and fruit in the evening.

When you are buying wholemeal bread and rolls, try the squeeze test. Take the loaf lengthways between both palms of your hands and give it a gentle squeeze. If it compresses easily, don't buy it. As a general rule, the denser the loaf, the more fibre it contains and, consequently, the better it is for you.

Put wholemeal bread at the top of your shopping list and eat it at every meal. Try to find

71

a local bakery where you can buy it fresh every day – alternatively, you can make it yourself. Wholemeal bread has a wonderful texture and a nutty, interesting taste. You can choose from a good selection of mixed-grain breads such as granary, sesame, oatbran, and rye. Each has a distinctive flavour of its own. You could also try wholemeal pitta bread, which is delicious with salads and dips.

Vitamins

The vitamins and minerals contained within the foods that you eat as part of a healthy, balanced diet are essential pre-conceptually and during pregnancy to ensure the healthy development of the baby.

It is not necessary to take vitamin or mineral supplements, provided that you eat regularly and healthily, choosing food from all four food groups described on pages 70–1.

Some vitamins and minerals are hazardous in overdose, and a well-balanced diet is far preferable to taking synthetic supplements. A varied and balanced diet of wholefoods – those that are in their natural unprocessed state – should ensure that you receive a sufficient level of all the vitamins you need.

It is impossible to achieve the right balance of vitamins from supplements alone, and healthy food is the only way to obtain all the other essential nutrients.

The only supplement that is worth taking is folic acid (see opposite), which is part of the B vitamin complex, but it is possible to obtain this from your diet as long as you eat plenty of green leafy vegetables every day.

vitamin A

What it does: builds up resistance to infection; good for teeth, skin, hair, and fingernails, and for the formation of the thyroid gland
Food source: oily fish, fish liver oils, milk, margarine, butter, eggs, organ meats, green and yellow vegetables, carrots, oranges, apricots

vitamin B1

What it does: good for digestion, growth, lactation, and resistance to illness
Food source: organ meats, brewer's yeast, whole grains, wheatgerm, nuts, pulses

vitamin B2 (riboflavin)

What it does: good for eyes and skin and for growth and development of the embryo
Food source: organ meats, brewer's yeast, whole grains, wheatgerm, green vegetables, milk, eggs

vitamin B3 (niacin)

What it does: builds brain cells and promotes resistance to infection

Food source: organ meats, brewer's yeast, whole grains, wheatgerm, green vegetables, fish, eggs, milk, nuts

vitamin B5 (pantothenic acid)
What it does: maintains red blood cells
Food source: organ meats, whole grains, wheatbran, eggs, cheese, nuts

vitamin B6 (pyridoxine)
What it does: promotes resistance to disease, is good for the nerves, and promotes the formation of healthy red blood cells
Food source: organ meats, meat, fish, brewer's yeast, whole grains, wheatgerm, vegetables, bananas, molasses, eggs, dairy products

vitamin B12
What it does: promotes the formation of healthy red blood cells; good for the baby's central nervous system
Food source: organ meats, red meat, eggs, milk, cheese, fish

folic acid (part of B complex, also sometimes called vitamin M)
What it does: helps cell division, which is essential for the baby's central nervous system; deficiency of folic acid has been linked with brain and spinal cord defects at birth, and women who have previously given birth to a baby with one of these defects (such as spina bifida) are now prescribed folic acid before conception
Food source: green leafy vegetables, lamb's liver, walnuts

vitamin C (ascorbic acid)
What it does: helps resistance to infection, promotes the absorption of iron, encourages the development of a healthy placenta
Food source: fresh fruits, particularly citrus fruits and strawberries, all fresh vegetables, particularly potatoes, green peppers, and tomatoes

vitamin D (calciferol)
What it does: encourages the absorption of calcium and promotes the formation of strong bones
Food source: oily fish, fish liver oils, liver, milk, eggs, butter

vitamin E
What it does: promotes the formation of healthy cells
Food source: most foods, particularly wheatgerm, vegetable oils, fish, green leafy vegetables, whole grains and pulses

vitamin K
What it does: enhances the ability of blood to coagulate
Food source: green leafy vegetables

Minerals

Calcium, iron, and zinc are the three minerals that are important both pre-conceptually and during pregnancy.

Calcium

It is important to make sure that you are obtaining sufficient calcium pre-conceptually because once you are pregnant, the baby will deplete your reserves of calcium.

Calcium is important for the healthy formation of your baby's teeth and bones, which begin to form from around weeks 4–6. Calcium is better absorbed during pregnancy than at other times, and your baby is unlikely to go short. The baby will take what calcium he or she needs, but this may leave you deficient for your own teeth and bones.

Your calcium requirement therefore increases as your baby grows during pregnancy. By week 25, your requirement will have more than doubled, so you will need to ensure that you are eating and drinking plenty of calcium-rich foods.

Calcium supplements are useful for women who never drink milk, either because they are allergic to it or because they simply don't like it. You can take up to 1200mg of calcium supplements a day, though if you are eating well, 600mg should be enough.

Calcium is not absorbed efficiently without vitamin D. This vitamin is found in milk, butter, and eggs. Most importantly, though, the body will manufacture its own vitamin D with the help of exposure to the sun. You can take vitamin D in the form of halibut oil capsules, which also contain vitamin A, but you must take care not to

CALCIUM-RICH FOODS INCLUDE

milk • yoghurt • leafy green vegetables • nuts • pulses • sesame seeds • sardines

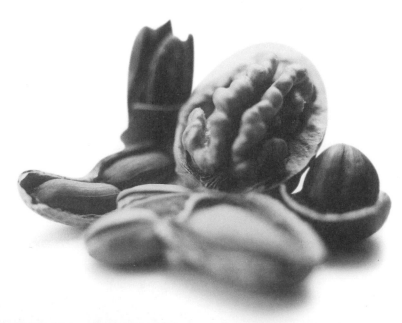

overdo your intake of vitamin A, either pre-conceptually or while you are pregnant, as an excess of this vitamin during pregnancy can lead to birth defects.

Iron

As soon as you become pregnant, the large increase in the volume of blood in your body means that you will probably need almost twice as much iron as you did before you became pregnant. It is therefore a good idea to make sure that your iron reserves are adequate before you conceive.

Iron is necessary for the formation of red blood cells, which contain a substance called haemoglobin. If you don't have sufficient haemoglobin in your blood, insufficient oxygen may be carried to your baby, which will also result in your becoming very tired.

The baby will build up a supply of iron in his or her own liver, which will last for several months after the birth. This is very important because milk – the baby's diet for several months – contains virtually no iron.

The body does not absorb iron very easily. Vitamin C, which is present in fresh fruit and vegetables, helps the body to absorb iron. Antacid medicines, on the other hand, hinder the absorption of iron, and it is therefore best to avoid them.

Many women are routinely given iron tablets in the second and third trimesters of their pregnancy. This is not usually necessary if you are eating a balanced diet containing many iron-rich foods.

If you are at all worried about your intake of iron once you become pregnant, you should talk to your medical practitioner during your antenatal check-ups.

Vegetarians and vegans are advised to take iron supplements during pregnancy. An excellent herbal iron tonic is also available at health food stores.

Zinc

It is well worth making sure you are obtaining sufficient zinc pre-conceptually, because the body's levels of zinc often fall dramatically during pregnancy – by as much as 30 per cent. There is also some evidence to suggest that an inadequate intake of zinc during pregnancy can result in a small baby or a premature birth.

75

IRON-RICH FOODS INCLUDE

red meat • liver • dark molasses whole grains • egg yolk • pulses dark green leafy vegetables • raisins prunes • brewer's yeast • nuts

ZINC-RICH FOODS INCLUDE

oily fish • wheatgerm • brewer's yeast • oysters • meat • walnuts • eggs pumpkin seeds • molasses • onions • nuts • peas • beans

Your healthy living plan: what to avoid

With so many pollutants and toxins present in the air you breathe, emissions from industrial sites and road traffic, and chemical residues in rivers and crops, it is vital to take care that the food you eat is safe and wholesome.

On the one hand, you can ensure that you follow a healthy diet as part of pre-conceptual care, and on the other hand, you can avoid all those foods that are either without nutritional value or are positively harmful. You should also be extra careful to avoid other hazards that could contaminate your food.

Listeriosis

Listeriosis is an infection caused by bacteria called Listeria monocytogenes and, if caught by a woman during pregnancy, it can result in miscarriage, stillbirth, or severe illness in the newborn baby.

In 1990, listeriosis affected 1 in 30,000 births in Britain. High levels of listeria have been found in foods such as some cheeses, so it may be advisable to avoid these (see opposite). Otherwise, be sure that foods are "in date" and are kept in a refrigerator where the temperature is maintained at under 5 degrees C (use a thermometer to check that this is the case).

Campylobacter pylori

This is the chief cause of food poisoning and far outweighs the other causes, including listeria and E. coli. This bacterium is predominantly found in raw meat, poultry, wild birds, and unpasteurized milk.

Toxoplasmosis

Toxoplasmosis is an infection caused by a parasite. It is usually harmless in adults and the chances of catching it are about 10 per cent for every 10 years you live. There are very few symptoms (usually no worse than mild flu), and it cannot be passed from person to person. However, if toxoplasmosis is caught by a woman during pregnancy, it can cause miscarriage or damage to her unborn baby. The infection may lead to damage to the brain. About 550 babies a year are born with the infection in the UK, of whom 10 per cent will be severely affected.

A test can be carried out in pregnancy to detect antibodies to toxoplasmosis (similar to the test for rubella). This will establish whether or not you are immune. Unfortunately, the test itself is not perfect and can sometimes provide borderline results, leading to more questions than answers.

If you have already been infected and are immune, toxoplasmosis will not affect any future pregnancies.

The parasite lives in cats for about three weeks, but cats' faeces can remain infectious for up to 18 months, so careful hygiene is necessary (see page 67).

During pregnancy, because of the threat of toxoplasmosis affecting the unborn baby, the general food hygiene measures described on page 68 should be observed.

Fresh fruit, vegetables, and lettuce are all potential sources of toxoplasmosis infection and should be thoroughly washed under running water before they are eaten.

Toxoplasmosis is also caught from the soil and from raw meat (see page 67).

FOODS THAT MAY CONTAIN HIGH LEVELS OF LISTERIA

unpasteurized milk • pâté made from meat, fish, or vegetables • mould-ripened and blue-veined cheeses • soft-whip ice cream from ice cream machines • pre-cooked poultry and cook-chill meals, unless thoroughly reheated • prepared salads, unless washed thoroughly

FOODS TO AVOID BEFORE AND DURING PREGNANCY

The following list includes the food and drinks that are best avoided as part of your pre-conceptual care and healthy living package.

Some of these foods have an associated risk factor, while others are lacking in nutritional value and are better replaced in your diet by the healthy, wholesome foods listed on pages 70–71.

alcohol • biscuits • cakes • cheeses (soft, blue-vein and soft unpasteurized goat and sheep's cheeses, because of the risk of listeriosis) • chocolate • coffee • colas • cream • eggs, raw or lightly cooked (because of the risk of salmonella) • food additives and colourants • fried foods • junk food • liver and liver products (such as pâté and liver sausage) • poultry, undercooked (because of the risk of salmonella) • pre-cooked, pre-packaged convenience foods • raw beef (steak tartare, rare beef, and rare hamburgers) • red meat (once a week is ample for health) • salt added to food • salty snacks such as crisps and spicy tortilla chips, salted nuts • shellfish, raw • smoke and tar from tobacco (the most damaging toxin of all) • sugar added to food, or any foods or snacks containing white sugar • sweetened drinks • sweets • takeaway meals • white processed bread

77

Detox guidelines

The many pollutants present in the environment make the routine of a regular detox highly appealing, but cleansing and detoxification programmes have a limited part to play in pre-conceptual care. Their chief role is one of eliminating toxins from the body, inducing relaxation and a sense of well-being. The benefits of a pre-conceptual detox are truly enjoyed when undertaken with your partner.

There is no need to buy any special products or supplements to use in a detox programme. Be wary of the unsubstantiated claims made for many products associated with detoxing which are available in health stores and pharmacies. For a successful detox, all you need is some time to focus on yourself and your partner.

Pick a day or a weekend for your detox. Start your day with a glass of water with a generous slice of lemon, which possesses good antiseptic and cleansing properties.

In order to boost your metabolism, eat a slice of plain wholemeal bread without butter or any other spread. This really wakes up the digestive system and starts the process of shifting long accumulated food deposits. It is important to keep the fire stoked, as it were, so that your metabolism is working at full power. One of the disadvantages of fasting is that the body's systems start to slow down and digestion becomes increasingly sluggish.

The next step in your detox day can be 30 minutes' brisk exercise taken with your partner. This could take the form of running or fast walking, for example. This exercise speeds up your circulatory system, which brings freshly oxygenated blood to all parts of the body and also assists in lymph drainage, an essential part of the elimination of toxins from the body.

After your exercise, drink a glass of water, followed by a glass of liquidized fruit or vegetables – both are excellent detoxifiers.

Next, you and your partner should dry brush your whole bodies in order to remove dead skin cells. Use exfoliating cream for your face, hands, feet, and elbows. Now take a bath or shower together.

Once your skin is supple from the warm water and clean through your dry brushing routine, do an aromatic steam inhalation in order to speed up facial cleansing.

Once you have completed these steps, drink two glasses of water to help flush out accumulated toxins. You and your partner may like to give one another a full body massage, which greatly assists in lymphatic drainage.

Drinking plenty of water – about two litres every day – is central to a detox programme. Keeping up your fluid intake is vital even when you are not detoxing.

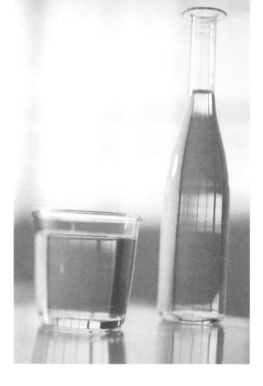

DETOX TIPS

- *Drink nothing but water (with or without a slice of fresh lemon) – about a couple of litres during the course of the day. Have a large bottle for each of you on hand so that you can monitor how much you have drunk*

- *Exercise vigorously every two or three hours with stretch and tone exercises in between*

- *Massage, steam inhalation, exfoliation, and salt rub (you can also take saunas and whirlpool baths)*

- *Eat lightly every two or three hours from your favourite fibre-rich foods*

- *Take time out to relax, perhaps through meditation (see page 126) or yoga (see pages 88–91)*

- *Cleanse and moisturize each other's skin with essential aromatic oils (see pages 104–8)*

- *After a warm and sensuous bath, go to bed an hour or two earlier than usual – without newspapers, television, or laptop*

FASTING

Fasting is not recommended for anyone, and particularly not for anyone who is hoping to become or is already pregnant.

As part of your detox day, play a game of tennis or whichever exercise appeals to you, followed by another glass of water.

After your exercise, you might like to give one another a salt rub in the bath to help slough off dead skin and speed up the detox process. Waste products are excreted partly through the skin and therefore massage, exfoliation, and salt rubs are important in keeping the pores clean and healthy.

Remember to keep drinking lots of water and eat small quantities of detoxifying foods every couple of hours. Suitable foods include fresh uncooked vegetables and fruit, vegetable soups, liquidized vegetable drinks, and wholemeal bread.

Stretch and tone exercises and skipping routines will tone up your cardiovascular fitness, and, again, help to eliminate toxins from your body.

Exercise

Exercising as part of your pre-conceptual care and care during pregnancy will help maintain optimum fitness of all the systems of the body, especially the reproductive system. You will also benefit from achieving the feel-good factor that good exercise induces.

The release of freshly oxygenated blood around the body repairs and renews all the cells of the body, including those of the reproductive system. Regular exercise boosts the cardiovascular system, strengthening the lungs and heart and improving the circulation, to help in this vital process.

The feel-good factor

The release of endorphins – the so-called "feel-good" hormones – that is induced by exercise helps to banish the stresses of everyday life and relieve fatigue. When you are feeling physically fit, you will find you are able to manage all your everyday tasks, at work and at home, with increased vitality and reduced stress. You are much less likely to lose your temper when you are put under pressure, less likely to make mistakes, and more likely to derive pleasure and fulfilment from your work, from your family life and from your friendships.

Being fit helps to prevent heart disease, control blood pressure, improve diabetes, control the weight, develop body strength, alleviate arthritis, improve mobility, reduce breathlessness on exertion, prevent osteoporosis, fight off depression and feelings of apathy, and reduce the risk of a stroke.

HOW FIT ARE YOU?

- *The lift's broken down and walking up four flights of stairs makes you out of breath*
- *You are out of breath running across platforms for a train*
- *You haven't won a tennis/squash/ badminton match in ages*
- *You drive everywhere*
- *You are gaining a little weight every year, year after year*
- *You become tired more easily and quickly than you used to*

Sounds familiar? You are probably not as fit as you would like to be or as fit as you could be.

80

FITNESS AIMS

General fitness comprises the following:

muscular strength • muscular endurance • cardiovascular endurance • flexibility • speed • power

---

Why fitness is important

Doctors and other experts now recognize, unequivocally, that exercise and activity are good for us, both mentally and physically. They also know that many people are resistant to the idea of exercise for a variety of reasons:

"I can't find the time."

"It's all I can do, when I get home, to get the supper and collapse in front of the TV."

"I'm always on my feet anyway – I certainly don't need to do any more."

The time factor

Finding the time to exercise depends a lot upon your personal motivation. If you really want to become fit (or fitter still), you will always find the time even if it means deciding that sheets, pillowcases, towels, and T-shirts do not need to be ironed, or videoing your favourite TV programme in order to watch it later, or getting up half an hour earlier in the morning.

Take a good look at how you spend your evenings. Do you find time to watch something on TV when you could be exercising? Do you chat on the telephone even though you know you are going to see that person at the weekend? What in your evenings or weekends can be relinquished to make space for half an hour's physical activity each day?

The fatigue factor

It is well known that exercise provides you with more energy rather than less. However, no one will believe it until they have actually done it. Try just once going for a walk or a swim after work, and see how much better you feel. You will also find that your quality of sleep is improved, so that you feel better when you wake up the next morning. Alternatively, go for a walk or a swim before work. Getting up half an hour earlier each morning reaps rich rewards.

What sort of exercise

Many experts believe that walking and swimming are the two best possible forms of exercise to undertake on a regular basis for optimum general fitness. They are both rhythmic and sustained, and they both use several sets of muscles. Swimming uses nearly all the muscles of the body and is particularly suitable if you are overweight, in that the weight of the body is borne by the water. Walking is a valuable form of exercise and one that can easily be incorporated into your way of life.

You don't even need to go out of the house to achieve fitness: if the only way that you can

OVERALL FITNESS

In order to achieve fitness in all its dimensions – such as strength, endurance, flexibility, speed, and power, you need a good mix of different types of exercise. Choose from some of the following exercises:

aerobics class • aquaerobics class • cycling • dance class • gym • pelvic-floor exercises • skipping • stretch and tone class • swimming • walking • yoga

manage 30 minutes of moderately brisk activity each day is to set aside half an hour at home, then choose from step exercises, walking up and downstairs, exercising with weights, skipping, sit-ups, aerobics (to video or music), or stretch and tone exercises.

How long should I exercise?

If you are exercising regularly, 30 minutes a day, three days a week of moderately brisk activity is sufficient to build and maintain fitness. As your fitness levels increase, you will be able to achieve more and more in your daily half an hour.

When you have achieved your desired level of fitness, brisk activity 30 minutes a day, three days a week, will maintain your fitness and continue to improve your general muscle tone.

What matters most is the regularity of the exercise you undertake, rather than whether you carry it out on three or five days of the week.

Feeling the benefits

The effects of exercise on the body are a powerful force in keeping the spirits up. In the last two decades of the 20th century, more and more research attested to the benefits of the feel-good hormones (the endorphins), which are released during vigorous exercise.

You will enjoy increased energy levels when you exercise regularly. Exercise causes blood sugar to rise and you are less likely to lack energy, and less likely to feel hungry and need to snack on carbohydrates.

The heart, the most important muscle of the body, grows stronger and larger with exercise and can therefore pump more oxygenated blood to the muscles with less effort and fewer beats. This reduces strain on the heart.

When you are unfit, the heart has to work harder and beat much faster to pump the required amount of blood through the system. When your system is sluggish, waste products stay in the body for longer. This can lead to the formation of deposits in the arteries, and these in turn can impede the flow of freshly oxygenated blood to all parts of the body. The heart has then to work even harder to overcome this resistance and, consequently, blood pressure is raised and even more strain is put

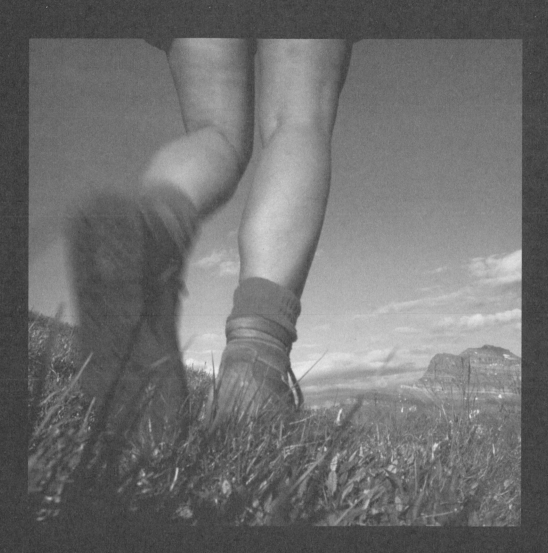

on your body. Regular exercise should be regarded as a lifestyle choice – when you make it a regular part of your life you will feel the benefits and never look back!

Exercise is vital for toxic waste to be eliminated from the body. This elimination

Walking is one of the best forms of exercise to do on a regular basis. It uses several sets of muscles and can easily be included in your daily routine. Try walking up the escalator, getting off your bus one stop early and walking the rest of the way, and going for a short walk at lunchtimes. You will feel the difference within a short period of time.

84

EXERCISE TIPS

- *Drink at least eight glasses of water every day and more when you are exercising. Drink a glass before you start and another when you finish, and sip water throughout as necessary. Do not become dehydrated.*

- *Wear loose, comfortable clothing.*

- *Wear appropriate footwear for your chosen exercise or sport.*

- *Stop if you have any unexplained aches and pains.*

- *When you have cooled down after exercise, take a warm shower or bath to relax fully and to stretch out the muscles you have just worked.*

- *Build up your exercise routine gradually. It may take a few weeks to see a real improvement as your body adjusts to regular exercise. Only by taking it gradually will you become stronger and fitter. You will then be able to do more and sustain a higher level of fitness than before.*

- *Take a rest from exercise if you have a cold or infection.*

- *Avoid exercising in very hot weather as it is easy to become dehydrated.*

- *Remember that your body needs time to rest and recuperate. Don't squeeze all your exercise into the weekend and do nothing during the week. This will only put a strain on a body that has been relatively inactive for the previous five days.*

occurs principally through urination, defecation, and sweating. The whole body is stimulated through regular sustained exercise to function more efficiently and more quickly, so that waste products are excreted without delay and all the systems of the body – including the reproductive system – are able to function more efficiently.

You may experience a few aches and pains in the first few days of exercise as your tired muscles become accustomed to new challenges. Muscles may ache, but it will not take them long to get used to your new routine.

Exercise routines

Certain routines should become an integral part of your exercise programme. These include remembering to drink plenty of water before and after exercise, and doing warming up and cooling down exercises every time you start and stop exercising.

Always warm your body up for about 5 minutes to stretch the muscles and make them more flexible. This allows your body temperature to rise gradually and promotes a better blood supply to the working muscles for a more effective workout.

When you complete your workout, spend another 5 minutes going through the same set of exercises you used for your warm-up. This time you are doing them to allow your body to cool down. You need to bring your heart rate down gradually, and stretch your muscles now, while they are warm and supple, so that they don't stiffen up again. A few gentle warm-up exercises are included here.

Side steps

Stand with your feet apart. Move your right leg to the right, then close your left foot up to your right foot. Take another large sideways step with your right foot again, and join up with the left.

Now take one step to the left with your left foot. Bring your right foot behind the left foot. Take another step to the left with the left foot. Now take the right foot to join the left foot. Repeat five times. Repeat the sequence, starting by stepping to the left this time, and repeat five times.

Knee bends

Place your feet at about hip distance apart and, keeping your back straight and upright and your heels on the floor, bend your knees and lower your bottom slightly, then stand up straight. Repeat ten times.

Marching, low knees

This exercise consists simply of marching on the spot. Raise each foot in turn slightly from the floor and put it back again. You should bend your knees only slightly. Do not lift your feet too high as this is a low-impact exercise designed to reduce strain on your joints. March on the spot for about a minute.

Shoulder circles, shrugs

Push your left shoulder forward slowly until you feel the stretch in the muscles at the back of your shoulder. Push your shoulder back this time, again until you feel the muscles at the back of it stretching. Do each movement five times, then repeat the sequence with your right shoulder. Stand relaxed and shrug your shoulders up to your neck and back down. Repeat this ten times.

Exercise as part of your day

See how much additional physical exercise you can incorporate into your normal daily life. Always take the stairs rather than a lift. Get off the bus a couple of stops before your destination and walk the rest of the way. Walk up the escalator rather than just standing and letting it carry you. Don't take the car if you are going only a short distance. Park your car a mile away from your home. Park your car at the far end of the supermarket car park. Go for a short brisk walk each lunchtime. Run up and down the stairs at home.

Over a period of time, all these small activities add up to more exercise in your life and a feeling of growing physical power and delight in the strength and endurance of your body. A growing awareness of your own physicality is an important element of your preparation and care before you become pregnant and during your pregnancy.

85

Alexander Technique

The Alexander Technique aims to improve your health through better posture. It is particularly useful as part of your pre-conceptual care as it allows the reproductive system to function at its best without postural hindrance. It is also valuable during pregnancy in order to alleviate the strains and stresses on your back imposed by the growing baby.

The Alexander Technique has been called a method of posture training, but it goes much further than this. It is based on the belief that incorrect patterns of movement, to which we become habituated, hamper the natural functions of the body and set up a situation where disease can develop.

Posture and balance

It may be more accurate to describe Alexander Technique as a method through which body and mind are harmonized. It is a re-education of the whole self towards balance and freedom in movement and thought.

Its founder, the actor F. Matthias Alexander, was born in Tasmania in 1869. He found himself habitually losing his voice when he was on stage, but eventually discovered that he could cure the problem by improving his posture. This simple discovery became the starting point of an entire system of retraining the body's movements and positions, and today there are Alexander Technique schools and training centres all over the world.

Devotees claim that the technique can help improve your health, both physical and mental, and can, as a result, make you more resistant to stress. It is claimed to have been successful in treating conditions such as depression, anxiety, headaches, hypertension, infertility, respiratory problems, exhaustion, arthritis, back trouble, and digestive disorders.

Before and during pregnancy

The Alexander Technique will help you to get in touch with your body and to become more sensitive to its demands.

It will help you to adapt your ways of moving as you change shape during pregnancy, so that you do not make things unnecessarily uncomfortable for yourself, or hazardous for your baby. In particular, it will help you to use your body correctly so that backache – a problem that has for so long been assumed to be an inevitable part of pregnancy – may be entirely avoided.

The Alexander Technique will help you prepare for the birth, thus making it as natural a process as possible. It teaches you to stay upright, squatting, during labour, and to move in a relaxed way by consciously releasing tension. Tension increases pain, and tension itself may result as an unthinking reaction to pain. If you are relaxed, you can learn to cope with the pain and to allow the natural process of labour to take its course.

The lesson

The Alexander Technique is taught on a one-to-one basis in a series of lessons. When you begin, the teacher will watch how you use your body. Young children move naturally, but most people develop bad habits as they get older, and these, by adulthood, have usually become firmly ingrained.

The teacher's aim is to show you how you can change these bad habits and regain the ability to use your muscles with the minimum effort and the maximum efficiency. In this way, the teacher will retrain you to perform a whole range of everyday tasks – opening a door, getting in and out of a chair, getting in and out of the car, sitting at a desk, even answering the telephone.

Natural positions

The teacher does all this by gently manipulating your body, while you are standing, sitting, or lying down, into more natural positions. He or she will also give verbal instructions to help you become more aware of your posture and to help the natural mechanisms of poise to function more freely. Gradually, as you practise better posture, you will be able to release inbuilt tensions and learn to use your body correctly. The teacher will use no force, just a series of gentle manipulations and subtle adjustments.

A lesson lasts about 30–45 minutes. It is usual to have a course of 30 lessons, after which you should be able to continue on your own. Practitioners of the Alexander Technique are called teachers, not therapists, and the people they teach are called pupils, not patients.

Practising the technique

Bad postural habits are usually so ingrained that they have come to feel entirely natural and it is virtually impossible, without help, to recognize what you are doing wrong. But once you understand the principles of the Alexander Technique you may be able to see when your posture is slouched or awkward, simply by watching yourself in the mirror, which is what Alexander himself did. Because the principles are applied to everyday tasks, you can continually develop and reinforce your new awareness of your body's movements.

Yoga

This ancient system of postures from India is perhaps the foremost relaxing exercise of all. It is supremely suited for use as part of your pre-conceptual package, during pregnancy, and in the early stages of labour.

"Yoga" is a Sanskrit word meaning, literally, "yoke" or "union". This refers to the union between physical, mental, and spiritual training that lies at the heart of yoga. It is much more than just an exercise. It is a Hindu philosophy that aims to achieve a state of physical and spiritual well-being through certain physical exercises and postures.

One of the most important aims of yoga is to raise the level of primal energy, known as the *kundalini shakti*, which is contained in the base centre or *muladhara chakra* (energy centre), situated at the end of the coccyx at the base of the spine. Raising this energy level will bring about a state of enlightenment and realization.

There are five main types of yoga, all of which are accepted by the schools of Indian philosophy. These are:

- karma yoga
- jnana yoga
- bhakti yoga
- raja yoga
- hatha yoga

Broadly speaking, hatha yoga is the basis of the modern practice of yoga in the West and is the system of yoga that aims to achieve health and longevity. In India, yoga is a profoundly religious system of philosophy, which has existed for thousands of years. In the West, many people take up yoga largely for the reason that it teaches relaxation, as well as increasing the body's mobility and flexibility.

The postures (asanas) that yoga teaches reduce stress, make you sleep better, and leave you feeling calm, relaxed, and with a clear, untroubled mind. In this way, yoga promotes both inner and outer harmony. The postures involve a deliberate stretching and releasing of the muscles. They are done slowly and held for a few minutes, which helps to develop an awareness of the body, and of its tensions, both inner and outer.

Yoga has gained greatly in popularity, not just as an exercise but as a therapy in the management of certain ailments, particularly of stress and stress-related problems. It is recommended, for example, for anxiety and asthma, because it frees the chest and makes

88

breathing easier, and it is also good for alleviating heart conditions.

One of the reasons that yoga is so good for asthma sufferers is that breathing plays such an important part in its postures. According to the philosophy of yoga, breath embodies the individual's life force, or *prana*. Although breathing is usually an unconscious action, it is possible to become aware of it and to control it. In this way, it can have an important effect on a person's well-being.

Yoga can be practised by people of both sexes and all ages, from the very young to the elderly. It is a particularly suitable form of exercise for women who are intending to become pregnant because it is very gentle.

When you start, it is best to learn yoga from a qualified teacher and then you can practise the postures at home. Yoga is most beneficial if it is done regularly – ideally, daily, perhaps for just 15–20 minutes.

Before and during pregnancy

Relaxation is very important in the pre-conceptual phase and during pregnancy, and yoga is one of the best ways of training yourself consciously to relax.

When you are properly relaxed, there are a number of changes that take place in your body. The heart rate decreases and, because your heart is pumping blood at a slower rate, you begin to feel your whole body slowing down.

Your levels of blood sugar and blood fat, which automatically increase in response to stress, will start to return to a healthy level.

When you are pregnant, it is important to tell your yoga teacher, and to advise him or her of any previous problems or miscarriages you have experienced. It is not advisable to start yoga for the first time during your pregnancy without a teacher. There are some teachers who specialize in yoga for pregnancy.

You should be careful to do only those postures in which the abdomen is well extended, so as to create space for the growing baby. You should feel no discomfort or strain, and, if you do, you should come out of the asana.

If you are already experienced in yoga, you should keep it up throughout your pregnancy. Your body secretes a hormone at this time known as "relaxin", which makes you even softer and bendier than usual, so you may notice an improvement in your asanas. Sitting poses are particularly good because they help to open up the pelvis before the birth.

Standing poses are also recommended, because they strengthen the legs, which helps you to carry the extra weight of the baby. It is important to listen to your body at all times – only you can really judge what you are capable of doing and how best to adapt your asanas as you grow bigger.

Some of the asanas that are of particular benefit to pregnant and conceiving women are described here.

Squatting

Pregnant women should practise squatting often – not only when they are doing these yoga postures but at regular times throughout the day. Squatting regularly strengthens the legs and the perineum, so it is a very good preparation for delivery.

Becoming accustomed to feeling comfortable in this position will help you during labour because it is such an effective position in which to deliver.

1 With your feet apart, squat with your knees apart and your heels on the floor. Hold your knees with your arms. This position should feel quite comfortable. You should stay in a squatting posture until the legs become warm. You might not get your heels on the floor at first, in which case you might find it helpful to support the buttocks on a folded blanket, but with practice it will become easier.

2 While you are in a squatting position, stretch the back by pulling your head forward and down, feeling the stretch down the neck and upper back.

3 To come out of this posture, slowly raise the buttocks so that the legs straighten. Let the upper body hang from the hips, with the arms loose. Hold this position for a moment, then stand up slowly, lifting the head last. Take a deep, cleansing, diaphragmatic breath.

Standing

This involves two poses: one standing tense, one standing relaxed. These strengthen and tone the muscles, and then release the tension.

1 Stand with the pelvis tucked under, ankles together, and feet at about 90 degrees. As you breathe in, tighten the legs, buttocks, arms, and abdomen. Hold this posture for a minute or two, breathing normally.

2 Release the posture with an outbreath.

Repeat this posture two or three times.

Upper thigh and pelvic stretch

This posture strengthens the pelvis and the upper thighs, so it is a useful exercise in preparation for labour.

1 Sit on the floor, bend the knees out to the sides and draw the heels in towards the groin. Join the soles of the feet together.

2 Hold the ankles and bring the feet close to the perineum. Press the feet lightly together. Keep the knees level.

3 Place your fingertips on the floor behind the hips and stretch the back of the body upwards.

Change legs and repeat. Take a deep, cleansing breath.

Leg raises

These strengthen and tone the abdomen, pelvic, and leg muscles. They relieve tension, especially if you have any leg discomfort.

1 Lie down on your back and breathe in. You can put a book or cushion under your head if you wish. Use your hands to cushion your coccyx bone. As you breathe out, slowly raise one leg. Lower the leg as you breathe in.

2 Raise the other leg as you breathe out.

3 Continue in this way, raising and lowering each leg in turn, for 2–3 minutes.

Cat posture

This posture relieves pressure of the fetus on the nerves and blood vessels of the lower pelvis and upper thighs. It also relieves backache and improves spinal flexibility.

1 Kneel and place your hands on the floor beneath your shoulders, shoulder width apart. Hands and knees should be square, and the body and head should be parallel to the floor.

2 As you breathe in, slowly arch the back. Spread the buttocks and raise the head and neck, keeping the face relaxed.

3 As you breathe out, tuck the pelvis under and lower your head.

Repeat this slowly and gently several times, alternating a concave spine with a curled-up one. Slowly build up your capacity to 50 times, and repeat the whole thing four or five times a day – on waking, before and after your nap, before dinner, and before going to bed. This can be done right up until you go into labour.

Finding a teacher

If you have individual yoga lessons, the teacher will advise you, and be able to tailor his or her routine to suit your individual case. If you go to a yoga class, it will not be possible to tailor the routine to suit you, and you will be expected to do more or less the same exercises as the other members of the class.

Some yoga classes are intended specifically for beginners, others for more advanced students. Choose a class that suits you. Tell the teacher that you are intending to become pregnant, along with any relevant details about former problems or miscarriages. This is important as there may be some poses that you should not attempt.

Once you have been taught the basics of yoga by a qualified teacher, it is quite possible to practise the postures at home. Most people prefer to keep on going to classes, however, in order to get expert supervision to make sure they are doing it properly. You can then supplement classes with additional asanas at home tailored to your needs.

Reflexology

Reflexology, also known as reflex zone therapy, is a therapy involving the massage of specific areas of the feet that are believed to relate to other parts of the body. Reflexology can be highly beneficial to the woman who is intending to become pregnant or the pregnant woman, and it is also known to have been effective in cases of infertility. It is also particularly helpful in alleviating a range of postnatal problems.

Reflexologists regard the feet as a "mirror" of the body – with the left foot relating to the left-hand side of the body, and the right foot to the right-hand side. Treatment may also be given via the hands in the same way.

The therapy is based on the belief that ill-health occurs when energy channels, which are thought to run throughout the body, become blocked, causing particular areas of damage. Massage of specific points on the soles of the feet is aimed at clearing those blockages, so that the energy can flow freely again to repair the damage to the system and thus heal the disease that has resulted. There are points on the feet and hands that correspond to all the organs, glands and parts of the body.

This kind of treatment was first practised in China some 5000 years ago, and it was also known in ancient Egypt some 4000 years ago. It was not introduced in the West until around 1913, when an American ear, nose, and throat consultant, Dr William Fitzgerald, developed a healing system called zone therapy. This involved applying pressure, either with the hands or with special instruments, to various parts of the body.

Complaints that have been successfully treated with reflexology include back pain, migraine, sinus problems, digestive troubles, arthritis, difficulties with periods, infertility, and stress. Treating the whole of the foot can have a general relaxing effect on the entire body.

Reflexologists also claim that they can sometimes predict a potential problem, which treatment can then pre-empt.

Before and during pregnancy

Reflexology can help in overcoming fertility problems in both sexes, but it has been found to be particularly effective for women who are having difficulty conceiving.

It is a surprisingly powerful form of therapy, which means that it may not always be suitable in the first three months of pregnancy. An experienced practitioner will, however, be able to advise you. After the initial stage of pregnancy, reflexology can help with relaxation and sleeping problems. It can also help to boost the immune system.

The course of treatment

On your first visit, the reflexologist will take a detailed case history. You will then lie in a comfortable reclining position, with your feet raised, and your shoes and socks removed. The therapist will first examine the condition of your feet, noting their general appearance, temperature, and colour. This examination will pick up tiny imbalances and congestions in the feet that indicate blockages of energy.

Before massage can begin, the reflexologist will massage talcum powder on to your feet, which will accustom you to having your feet handled. Surprisingly, reflexology does not tickle. He or she will then massage the feet, using the thumbs, and concentrating on any tender areas that indicate parts of the body may be out of balance.

The first treatment lasts for about an hour. A series of six to eight sessions, each one lasting about 30–40 minutes, is usual. Sessions may be weekly to start with, and may then be spread out at intervals of two or three weeks.

Detoxification

During a course of reflexology treatment, the body goes through a process of detoxification, which may manifest itself in aching joints, diarrhoea, or increased urination. This does not always happen, but, if it does, it should be regarded as a good sign and will not, in any case, last long.

Learning reflexology

The best results are obtained through consultation by a qualified practitioner, though it is possible for people to treat themselves, or each other, at home following the same techniques. Only relatively minor complaints, including back and neck pain, tension, sinus problems, catarrh and headaches, are suitable for unqualified treatment because of the powerful nature of this therapy.

You and your partner may choose to attend reflexology classes or lessons together so that you can learn the techniques and practise them upon one another at home.

The practitioner will work on the relevant meridian points in the feet, for both of you, for delay and blockage in your reproductive systems. After a joint consultation, you will probably both feel lighter and more relaxed in mood, more energetic, and free from stress and tensions. The treatment will help to counteract the anxiety that may be exacerbating the problem of delayed conception.

Massage

Massage is one of the oldest therapies, and can be found in every culture in the world. A perfect part of your pre-conceptual care, for both you and your partner to practise together, massage soothes away aches and pains and reduces tension.

94

Touch is a natural instinct to us, and without it people can become bad-tempered and depressed. We all need to be encouraged to touch each other more, and massage is the perfect way of doing this.

Even the simplest form of massage can be richly comforting, which can, in turn, have a profoundly beneficial effect on your sexual and reproductive health. Massage is known to improve circulation, relax muscles, help digestion, regulate the nervous systems, and speed up the elimination of waste products. These benefits, together with the psychological advantages of feeling cared for and pampered, soon produce a general feeling of well-being.

Massage is one of the oldest holistic therapies, in that it takes into account a person's whole being – physical, mental, and emotional. It is perhaps not surprising that Hippocrates, the ancient Greek physician who was hailed as the Father of Medicine, wrote as long ago as the 5th century BC: "The way to health is to have a scented bath and an oiled massage each day".

The principal aim of massage is to relax both mind and body and thus to relieve the stresses and strains of daily living. It is very successful in treating neck and back pain, particularly in people who spend the day hunched over a desk or sitting at the wheel of a car.

Success has also been claimed by therapists in dealing with many other problems, including circulatory disorders, heart conditions, high blood pressure, headaches, and insomnia. Athletes and sportspeople can gain enormously from massage, which eases stiffness and tones the muscles.

Before and during pregnancy

Gentle massage is highly beneficial to all conceiving and pregnant women. Many massage practitioners are experienced in treating pregnant women. A lot of them enjoy this work greatly, appreciating the tremendous benefits they are producing, as well as giving a much needed level of emotional support.

As well as being very relaxing, massage can alleviate some of the common complaints of pregnancy, including backache, insomnia, swollen legs, and even morning sickness.

Back massage

Backache is probably the most common complaint of all during pregnancy, and a back massage can do a lot to relieve the discomfort. As well as having a back massage done by a professional therapist, you can ask your partner to do this for you.

The best way is to sit astride a chair, facing its back, and lean on a cushion. Your partner should then use plenty of gentle stroking movements, which are very calming. He should not, however, apply deep pressure to the lower back, particularly during the first three months of pregnancy.

As well as easing your backache, this will give you a comforting sense of loving care and tenderness, which is in itself deeply beneficial.

Professional massage

You can visit the therapist's consulting rooms for a professional massage, though some therapists are happy to come to your home. Massage is usually given in a warm, quiet room, with the person being massaged lying on a firm, comfortable surface – preferably on a special massage table. The masseuse or masseur will oil his or her hands and spread the oil over the surface of the skin of the person being massaged. A light vegetable oil scented with essential oils is best.

A full-body massage usually lasts for about an hour, or an hour and a half if the face and head are being massaged at the same time.

Techniques

The massage techniques used in the West are usually those of Swedish massage. This relies on four basic massage movements: effleurage (stroking), petrissage (kneading), percussion (drumming), and friction (pressure).

These four movements, used individually or in combination, form the basis of any massage, although each practitioner will have his or her own favourite method and procedure.

Effleurage

Treatment almost always begins with effleurage. This consists of slow, rhythmic, stroking movements. The fingertips are used for light pressure, and the thumbs or knuckles for deeper pressure.

Petrissage

This consists of grasping handfuls of flesh, which are kneaded like dough, rolled, and released. Petrissage stimulates the circulation and helps to relax contracted muscles. It also helps to relieve any tendency towards cramp.

Percussion

These are short, fast, rhythmic movements, which are performed with the sides of the hands on any large, fleshy part of the body, such as the back, buttocks, shoulders, thighs, and waist. The movements should be brisk and light, and should not cause any pain, but are best avoided during pregnancy.

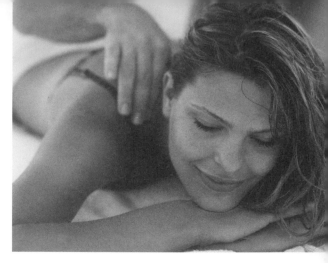

Friction

A series of small circular movements made by one or several fingers, the pads of the thumbs, or the heel of the hands, stimulates circulation and encourages joints to move more freely.

Self-massage

Self-massage may not be as enjoyable as being massaged by your partner but it can be soothing. You can use it to energize yourself during the day, or to unwind in the evening. It feels really good when done in the bath.

Shoulders

People's tensions tend to accumulate in their shoulders, causing aching shoulders, stiff necks, and headaches. The shoulders are a good place to begin your self-massage.

1 Stroke your right shoulder with your left hand. Stroke down the side of your neck, over

The caring touch of massage, administered by your partner or by a professional therapist, soothes away stresses and anxieties. It also has direct physical benefits, such as improving circulation.

your shoulder, and down the arm to your elbow. Repeat this sequence at least three times. Do the same on the other shoulder.

2 Using your fingertips, make small circular movements on either side of your spine, pressing quite firmly. Work up the neck to the base of the skull.

3 Knead your shoulder, squeezing and releasing the flesh on your shoulder and upper arm. Repeat on the other side.

Legs

Massage stimulates the circulation and soothes tired or swollen legs.

1 Sit on the floor, with your legs slightly bent. Rest the foot of one leg flat on the floor, and bend the knee. Stroke the whole leg with both hands. Start with the foot, then stroke up the calf, over the knee and finally up to the top of

MASSAGE SAFETY

There are a few conditions when massage is inappropriate. Do not have a massage when you have:

an infection • a high temperature • acute back pain, especially when the pain shoots down the arms or legs • a skin infection

the thigh. Do this about five or six times, then repeat the whole sequence on the other leg.

2 Knead the thigh using both hands alternately. Squeeze and release the flesh rhythmically. Repeat two or three times on each leg.

3 Stroke the thigh, working up from the knee with one hand following the other. Now repeat on the other leg.

4 Pummel each thigh with loosely clenched fists, concentrating on the front and outside to relieve any stiffness.

5 Using your fingertips, stroke around the kneecap. Then stroke gently behind the knee, up towards your thigh. Repeat on the other leg.

6 Knead the calf muscle using both hands, then stroke the area gently, with one hand following the other up the back of the leg. Repeat on the other leg.

Face

A face massage can relieve headaches, fatigue, and anxiety and tension. Use a good quality facial oil, which will prevent you dragging the skin.

1 Put your hands over your face, fingers on forehead, and heels of your hands on your chin. Leave the hands quite still for a minute or two, then slowly draw them out towards your ears.

Just feel the tension easing away. Repeat as many times as you like.

2 Pinch along your jawline, using the thumbs and knuckles of your forefingers of both hands. Begin just underneath the chin and work out towards the ears. Pinch near the bone so that you are not stretching the skin.

3 Using the backs of your hands alternately, slap them gently under your chin. This is a pleasantly stimulating movement, which will help prevent a double chin.

4 Stroke your hands, one after the other, up your forehead, working from the bridge of the nose to the hairline. Close your eyes as you do this and repeat as many times as you like.

5 Massage between your eyebrows. Place both index fingers on the bridge of your nose and stroke firmly, first upwards, and then across. This will help reduce any frown lines. Repeat as many times as you like.

6 Using the tips of your index and middle fingers, make circular movements all over the forehead. Press firmly but be careful not to drag the skin. Repeat as many times as you like.

7 Using your fingertips, stroke your forehead gently, working from the centre to your temples. Finally, press firmly against your temples.

Acupuncture

Acupuncture is an ancient Chinese system of medicine that uses needles to activate the body's energy channels, boost its natural functions – including the reproductive system – treat disease, bolster the immune system, promote the body's natural healing powers, and alleviate fatigue. You may find acupuncture useful both before and during your pregnancy, and as effective pain relief during labour.

98

Acupuncture is based on the ancient Chinese belief that the body is traversed by invisible energy channels, which are called "meridians". Each meridian is linked to a particular internal organ. Therefore, each organ of the body can be treated by stimulating the relevant meridian.

The system of acupuncture works on the theory that diseases can be treated by sticking needles into a patient's skin at particular points – known as acupuncture points – that lie along the meridians. The needles have the effect of unblocking the flow of energy or life force (called Qi or Ch'i) which runs through the meridians.

Any disorder, whether physical or emotional, is believed to alter the flow of energy through the meridians. It can make it flow too slowly or too fast, it can divert it to the wrong organ, or it may even block it completely. An acupuncturist aims to correct the flow and balance of energy – in other words, to unblock it, or make it flow faster or slower according to what is wrong with it – and cause it to return to its normal rate.

When an organ is suffering from disease, the acupuncture points often become tender. According to acupuncturists, the tenderness will disappear again as soon as the disease is treated, whether it is treated by conventional medicine or by acupuncture.

Acupuncture is a traditional Chinese therapy and an integral part of modern Chinese medicine. It regards the body as a balance between the two opposing yet complementary natural forces known as yin (the female force) and yang (the male force). Yin is passive and peaceful while yang is aggressive and confrontational. Yin represents dark, cold, moisture, and swelling. Yang represents light, heat, dryness, and tautness.

According to Chinese medicine, it is an imbalance between yin and yang in the body that results in disorder and disease. Too much yin, for example, can cause dull pains, chills, and fatigue, while too much yang can cause swelling, pain, headaches, and high blood pressure. The aim of acupuncture is to identify and treat any imbalance of yin and yang. According to ancient Chinese tradition, there were 365 acupuncture points on the body, but the Chinese have now described about 1000 of them in total.

The concept that lies at the root of acupuncture, with its strange blend of physical and metaphysical interpretation, can be difficult to understand, but there is a wealth of evidence that it works for a great many people, and can treat many different complaints.

In the West, acupuncture is used mostly to treat painful conditions like back pain, arthritis, and rheumatism. Research in America has shown that it can cause the body to produce natural pain-relieving substances, endorphins and encephalins, which dull the senses. It is not surprising, then, that acupuncture has been used successfully to relieve pain during childbirth, surgery, and dentistry.

Acupuncture has also been found to be helpful for people suffering from allergies, asthma, heart conditions, digestive problems, insomnia, headache and migraine, anxiety, stress, fatigue, backache and back disorders, skin conditions, and ulcers.

Before and during pregnancy

The Chinese believe that before a woman can conceive her body must be in perfect harmony. Only then can the flow of energy necessary for the formation of a healthy fetus be normal. Acupuncture achieves that perfect balance.

During pregnancy, the flow of energy through the body must be right in order for the fetus to develop in as healthy a way as possible. One of the most common complaints in pregnancy – morning sickness – can be greatly reduced by the use of acupuncture to correct any imbalance.

There are, however, certain points on each meridian that must be avoided during pregnancy. The points vary according to the stage of pregnancy you have reached. In general, they are the points that will stimulate the uterus, which is obviously not advisable in the early stages of pregnancy, as there is said to be a risk that it could lead to miscarriage.

There are many acupuncturists who specialize in treating pregnant women, and who are happy to accompany you to the hospital to provide you with a safe and natural method of pain relief during labour. Many acupuncturists who have done this observe that a woman in labour who is being treated with acupuncture never panics and succeeds in giving birth in a relaxed and easy way.

Nowadays, most hospitals are prepared for your delivery to be attended by an acupuncturist, but you should arrange this with them well in advance. Acupuncture can also be used to encourage the dilation of the cervix and to speed things along in labour – or to slow them down, depending on what is needed.

Consultation

The first thing an acupuncturist will do is to take a detailed case history. He or she will also ask you about your lifestyle, including diet, exercise, sleep patterns, and stress levels, and will then diagnose any complaints according to the ancient rules of Chinese diagnosis. Your tongue, your skin colouring and condition, your hair, your posture, and general demeanour will be examined. The sound of your breathing and your voice will also be noted.

You should tell the acupuncturist that you are intending to become pregnant.

The most important tool an acupuncturist has is pulse diagnosis, which enables him or her to tell the state of energy in the meridians simply by taking the patient's radial artery pulse at the wrist. This is known as "palpating". There are six pulses at each wrist, making 12 in total. Each represents one of the 12 main organs and functions of the body. The experienced acupuncturist can diagnose hundreds of different conditions by palpating. It is such a sensitive diagnostic tool that it can tell the skilled practitioner about your past illnesses, and even warn about any future illnesses.

These Chinese illustrations show the locations of the key acupuncture points along the meridians.

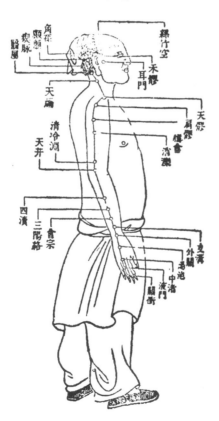

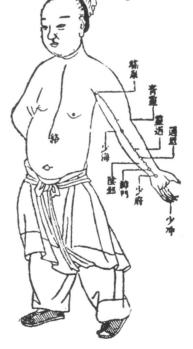

Once diagnosis has been made, the acupuncturist will then insert needles into acupuncture points in the body. The needles are very fine and are made of stainless steel. All needles must be disposable and presented in sealed sterilized packs, thus eliminating any possibility of transferring infection.

The insertion of the needles is usually quick, painless, and bloodless. The acupuncturist inserts them only about 6–12mm (¼–½in) deep and rotates them gently between finger and thumb, to draw or disperse energy from a point. You will probably experience a slight numbness or tingling sensation. The number of needles used varies. It can be as few as one or two, or as many as 15. Generally speaking, the more experienced the acupuncturist, the fewer the needles used. They can be left in for just a few minutes, or they can stay in for up to 30 minutes. This depends on the practitioner, the patient, and the condition being treated.

You may feel an improvement within the first four or five visits. Many patients report a feeling of lightness or buoyancy, or extreme relaxation after treatment. A complex problem, such as asthma, may require more sessions before there is any noticeable improvement. If there is absolutely no improvement after about eight sessions, acupuncture may not be the answer for that particular patient or complaint.

Occasionally, a patient may feel worse after the initial treatment. This is usually because the acupuncturist has over-stimulated the body's energies. In this case, fewer needles will probably be used, and for a shorter time, at the next session.

Many acupuncturists recommend a visit at each change of season, ie four times a year. This is believed to give the body an overall tune-up – rather like having a car serviced regularly.

Acupuncture cannot be done at home – either by you or by your partner – unless they are an acupuncturist. It must not be attempted by anyone who is not fully trained and qualified.

ACUPUNCTURE MERIDIANS

There are 14 meridians in total, each of which is named after the organ that it represents:

the heart • the small intestine • the bladder • the liver • the gallbladder • the lungs • the colon • the stomach • the spleen • the pericardium (not recognized in Western medicine), which controls the circulation • the "triple heater" or "warmer" (not recognized in Western medicine), which controls the function of the endocrine glands and acts as the body's thermostat • the "Ren" or "conception" (not recognized in Western medicine), which runs vertically up the centre of the front of the body • the "Du" or "governor" (not recognized in Western medicine), which also runs vertically up the centre of the back of the body

101

Acupressure

This ancient massage technique, which works on the acupuncture points along the body's meridians, is something you and your partner can practise and enjoy at home. It is also ideal for those who are attracted by the theory of acupuncture but shy away from the idea of needles.

You are using a form of acupressure whenever you rub a part of your body that hurts, or press your hands against your forehead to ease the pain of a headache.

Acupressure is thought to be a forerunner of acupuncture (see pages 98–101), although it uses firm thumb or fingertip pressure on points on the meridians, rather than inserting needles to stimulate the flow of Qi, or energy.

Like acupuncture, acupressure is used to balance the flow of energy through the meridians. There are various different schools of acupressure. The difference between them lies mainly in the various chosen combinations of pressure points and in the different degree of pressure applied.

Acupressure is largely concerned with relieving the symptoms of illness rather than dealing with the disease itself, although it is said to improve the body's own healing powers and thus to alleviate and prevent illness. It is thought to be a particularly appropriate form of treatment for people suffering from allergy, arthritis, asthma, back pain, circulatory problems, depression, digestive troubles, insomnia, migraine, and stress.

Some acupressure points must not be worked on during pregnancy. It is important to ask your therapist for advice about you as an individual: generalized advice cannot be given on this topic.

Only light pressure should be used on pregnant women. In general, the abdomen should be avoided, especially in the first three months of pregnancy.

One particularly common complaint in pregnancy is morning sickness, which responds well to acupressure.

To treat morning sickness

Make sure you are sitting comfortably and that you are warm. Then either massage these points yourself, or – better still – get your partner to do it for you.

Press with your thumb on a point about 5cm (2in) from the wrist on the inside of the arm. Apply pressure for between 5–10 minutes. The pressure may cause some minor discomfort, but no pain. Repeat the pressure as needed to ease the sickness. Work on both arms equally.

Seeing a practitioner

All acupressure practitioners begin by taking a case history, together with details of your lifestyle and diet. The therapist will also take your pulses for diagnosis, in the same way as is done in acupuncture (see page 100).

Pressure will then be applied to certain pressure points, depending on whether the therapist wants to stimulate or sedate the energy channels. Pressure may be applied in a variety of different ways, using the thumbs, fingertips, palms, knees, elbows, and even feet.

It is quite safe to use acupressure at home, particularly for common problems such as headache and nausea. However, you have to be careful, as there are some points that should not be stimulated pre-conceptually or during pregnancy. Although you can use acupressure on yourself, it is always better and more pleasant to get your partner to do it for you. A few sessions with a qualified therapist is the best way of learning exactly what to do.

Acupressure is used to balance the flow of energy through the meridians. It is said to boost the body's healing powers. Check with your therapist which points should not be massaged during pregnancy.

103

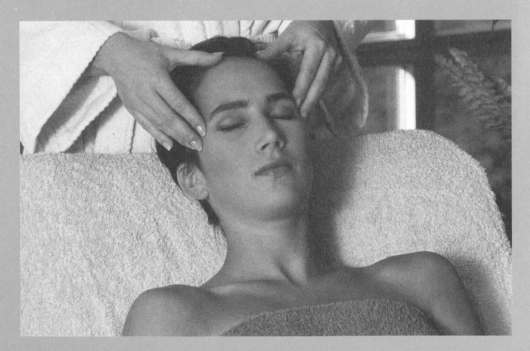

Aromatherapy

The art of treating illness using concentrated oils extracted from plants has been practised for generations. This is the most luxurious and pampering therapy, perfectly suited to a pre-conceptual package of care and throughout pregnancy.

Aromatherapists employ the medicinal benefits of oils extracted from plants, known as essential oils. When the oils are massaged into the body, they are absorbed in two ways: they are inhaled, and they are also absorbed through the skin. In this way, they are absorbed into the body fluids and bloodstream and can then set to work internally. They can also be added to baths or used for compresses.

The history of essential oils is a long and distinguished one. It was particularly important to the ancient Egyptians. When Tutankhamun's tomb was opened in 1922, a great many scent pots were discovered, which showed that aromatherapy was widely used by the wealthy people of the time. The Greeks used plant oils to heal wounds and to reduce inflammation, and the Romans also used plant oils widely.

It was not until the 16th century that the effects of plants on the human body were first investigated in Europe. It became a more and more fashionable practice over the years until, by the end of the 18th century, essential oils were widely used in medicine. Interest in their use declined during the 19th century, when it was regarded as strange and cranky, but interest was revived in the early part of the 20th century by a Frenchman, René-Maurice Gattefosse. Having burned his hand while conducting an experiment, he doused it in a dish of lavender oil which happened to be nearby. He was astounded by the speed with which his hand healed. It was Gattefosse who coined the name "aromatherapy" in the 1920s.

Aromatherapy is believed to be most helpful in treating long-term conditions, or recurring illnesses. Success has been claimed in treating stress and all related problems including depression, headaches, and insomnia. It is also good at treating pain-related problems, such as arthritis and cramp, and skin problems such as eczema and acne.

Doctors have become increasingly aware of its benefits, and scientists have confirmed the medicinal properties of many plants. They have proved, too, that the scent of the oils affects the cells in the nose, which send messages to the brain, and that the oils penetrate the skin. Further research is now being done to find out exactly how aromatherapy works.

Before and during pregnancy

The main and immediate effect of aromatherapy is relaxation, but there are many other benefits. It promotes general well-being and reduces fatigue. It relieves backache and tones the muscles, reducing aches and pains. Improved circulation means that there is less tendency to contract varicose veins or haemorrhoids. Fluid retention is reduced. Aromatherapy massage maintains the elasticity of the skin, helping to prevent stretch marks. Oils can be used to treat many of the minor problems of pregnancy, such as constipation, nausea, and heartburn.

It is important to be cautious in the use of essential oils when you are pregnant and you must tell your therapist if you are intending to become pregnant. All oils used in pregnancy should be diluted ½ to 1 per cent in a vegetable oil such as jojoba, sesame, or almond oil.

Many oils are not suitable for use at this time, as they will all be absorbed by the baby. Some have oxytocic properties, which stimulate the uterus. It is especially important to avoid these, particularly in the early months of pregnancy.

A consultation begins with a discussion of your general health and lifestyle. The practitioner selects the oils that are deemed to be best for you, taking into account both you as a person, and the nature of your problem. A full aromatherapy massage takes about an hour.

The therapist will probably also mix some oils for you to use at home, so you can continue the treatment yourself. Aromatherapy is easy to do at home, and there are many short courses available to teach you the basic principles. There are several methods by which you can treat yourself. These include:

Baths

Use for tension, backache, constipation, cystitis, aching muscles, insomnia, headaches, coughs, and colds. Add 4–6 drops of relaxing essential oil, such as lavender, to a hot bath. Lie back in the water and relax, breathing deeply, for 10–15 minutes.

Foot and hand baths

Use for localized aches and pains, and swelling. Add 4–6 drops of essential oil to a large bowl of hand-hot water. Soak the feet or hands for 10–15 minutes, topping up with warm water. Wrap feet or hands in a dry warm towel for a further 15 minutes.

Massage

Use for stress, skin problems, skin complaints, cramps, fluid retention, breathing difficulties, and to avoid stretchmarks. An essential oil, or a blend of oils, should be diluted for massage in a light vegetable oil, such as jojoba, sesame, or almond oil. During pregnancy it should always be diluted ½ to 1 per cent (or 5 drops of essential oil to 2 tablespoons of carrier oil), as oil absorbed by the skin will reach the baby. Apply diluted essential oils to the skin and massage in.

SAFETY: OILS TO AVOID

Do not use the following oils during pregnancy:

basil • cinnamon bark • clary sage • cedarwood • cypress • fennel • juniper • hyssop • marjoram/oregano • myrrh • nutmeg • parsley • peppermint • rosemary • sage • savory • thyme

Compresses

Use for bruises, varicose veins, haemorrhoids, sprains, burns, and scalds. Add 4–6 drops of essential oil to half a cup of water. Soak a piece of cotton wool in this, wring out, and place over the affected area. Place a warm towel over the compress and leave in place for at least 2 hours.

Inhalation

Use for tension, insomnia, nausea, breathing difficulties, coughs, and colds. Put 1–2 drops of essential oil on a tissue or handkerchief and inhale. Place the tissue or handkerchief on your pillow at night if you are having problems breathing. To make a steam inhalation, put 5–8 drops of essential oil in a bowl of hot water. Sit with your head above the bowl, and cover both head and bowl with a towel. Breathe deeply, closing your eyes to prevent irritation.

Essential oils are removed from plants in a complex extraction process that retains all the valuable properties of the oil.

Aromatherapy oils
Cajuput
Uses: Breathing difficulties, indigestion, toothache, earache, skin conditions, aches and pains, fatigue
Properties: Uplifting, soothing, antiseptic

Chamomile
Uses: Nausea, heartburn, indigestion, depression, headache, fluid retention, heartburn, cystitis, thrush, tension, stress
Properties: Refreshing, tonifying, relaxing, digestive, antiseptic, anti-fungal

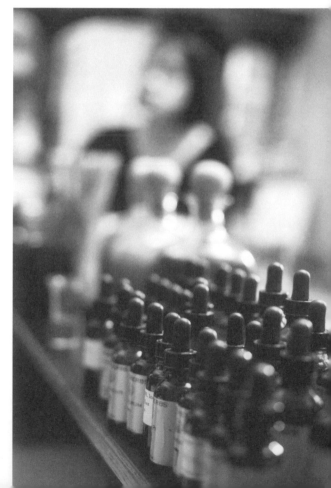

Eucalyptus

Uses: Fluid retention, muscular pain, headaches, infections, breathing difficulties, fever
Properties: Purifying, clears the air, antiseptic

Geranium

Uses: Cellulite, mastitis, pre-menstrual tension, diarrhoea, stress, tension, skin conditions, improves circulation, fluid retention
Properties: Tonifying, refreshing, relaxing, antiseptic, anti-fungal

Lavender

Uses: Depression, indigestion, insomnia, anxiety, aches and pains, fatigue, infections, high blood pressure, burns, skin conditions
Properties: Relaxing, refreshing, tonifying, antiseptic, anti-spasmodic, analgesic

Lemon

Uses: Circulatory problems, high blood pressure, skin conditions, infections
Properties: Tonifying, refreshing, fortifying, purifying, antiseptic

Neroli (orange blossom)

Uses: Anxiety, stress, insomnia, skin conditions
Properties: Relaxing, fortifying

Pine (*Pinus sylvestris*)

Uses: Infections, fluid retention, influenza, coughs and colds, catarrhal congestion
Properties: Refreshing, soothing, antiseptic, expectorant, decongestant

Sandalwood

Uses: Infections, fluid retention, skin conditions, respiratory infections
Properties: Soothing, refreshing, diuretic, stimulant, said to be aphrodisiac

Tangerine

Uses: Aches and pains, fluid retention, aids digestion, laxative
Properties: Tonifying, soothing, refreshing, harmonizes body and mind

107

DO'S AND DON'TS

- *Do buy high-quality oils from a specialist supplier of aromatherapy oils; the contents must be pure, undiluted essential oil, or an essential oil that has been diluted with a vegetable oil; pure oils are too strong for massage and must be diluted; pure oils can be used for other kinds of treatment*

- *Don't apply pure, undiluted oils directly to the skin*

- *Don't swallow essential oils*

Herbalism

There are hundreds of plants that, according to this ancient and worldwide system of medicine, can be used to prevent and cure a wide range of disorders and diseases. The power of herbal remedies should not be underestimated.

Herbal medicine consists of the preparation of plants in order to prescribe them to cure disease. Depending on the individual plant, different parts may be used – their roots, leaves, flowers, stem, or seeds – and they may be used fresh or dried.

Herbal preparations can be taken internally in the form of a tea or as tablets or capsules. Similarly, they can be applied externally in the form of an oil, a herbal bath, or a hand or foot bath; or they can be applied directly to the skin, in the form of a poultice, lotion, or ointment. In many cases, herbs can provide a safe, natural, and gentle alternative to medication.

also safe for most of us. The foremost value of herbal remedies is to treat everyday disorders.

Complaints that respond most commonly to herbal medicine include coughs and colds, catarrh, menstrual problems, fertility disorders, all kinds of aches and pains, including headaches, toothache, earache, and rheumatism, thrush, insomnia, skin conditions such as dandruff and acne, digestive problems such as diarrhoea and constipation, nervous disorders, and many minor injuries including burns, scalds, cuts, bruises, and insect bites. Herbal remedies are also used as preventative medicines.

The power of plants

Herbal medicines have been used throughout the world for many thousands of years. In modern times, they have been examined by scientists, who have discovered, in many cases, the scientific explanations for their uses.

By a combination of ancient tradition and modern science, it has been established that many herbal remedies are not only effective but

Before and during pregnancy

For centuries, herbal remedies have been used pre-conceptually, in pregnancy, as a preparation for childbirth, and during childbirth itself all over the world. Increasingly, women today are using herbs to enhance their general health. They are also using them to treat any problems that arise during pregnancy and to help ensure a safe and easy childbirth.

108

How to take herbal remedies

There are several ways in which you can take herbal remedies. The following can all be administered internally:

Infusions

These are made from the soft parts of the plant, such as the leaves, flowers, and stems. They are prepared in the same way as an ordinary cup of tea. The herbs are placed in a cup or a teapot, and boiling water is poured over them to draw out the medicinal constituents of the plant. The cup or pot is covered, and the mixture is left to infuse for 10–15 minutes before it is drunk.

If you are using dried herbs, one or two teaspoons of the herbs can be used per cupful of water, or 25g (1oz) of the herb to a pint of water. If you use fresh herbs, use two or three times the amount of herb to accommodate the extra water content of the plant.

A cupful of the infusion can be taken between three and six times daily. Herbs can be used singly or you can make up mixtures to suit your tastes.

Many aromatic herbs are available in teabags to make infusions, and are sold in healthfood stores, and they can be drunk daily as a healthy substitute for ordinary tea and coffee, which are really best avoided pre-conceptually and during pregnancy. You can also make your own teabags from dried herbs, using small muslin bags.

Decoctions

These are made from the harder, woody parts of the plant, such as the bark, wood, roots, nuts, and seeds. The pieces of bark, wood, or root are first broken up into tiny pieces or powdered so that their constituents can be more easily extracted by the water. They are placed in a saucepan, which may be either stainless steel or enamel but not aluminium, as some herbs may combine chemically with aluminium.

Cold water is poured over the herbs, in the ratio of 1–2 teaspoons per cupful of water or 25g to 50cl (1oz to 1 pint), plus a little more water to make up for any lost in the process. This is then brought to the boil, covered, and left to simmer for about 10 minutes. The resulting liquid is strained before use.

Tinctures

If you visit a herbal practitioner, you are most likely to be given your herbs in tincture form. Tinctures are fairly concentrated medicines made with water and alcohol to extract the constituents as well as preserving the preparation indefinitely once made.

The advantage of using tinctures is that they are easily administered and stored, and you only have to take small amounts at a time, which is especially attractive to those people who dislike some of the stronger-tasting remedies. The usual dose is one teaspoonful 1–3 times a day. You can also obtain tinctures from some herbal suppliers.

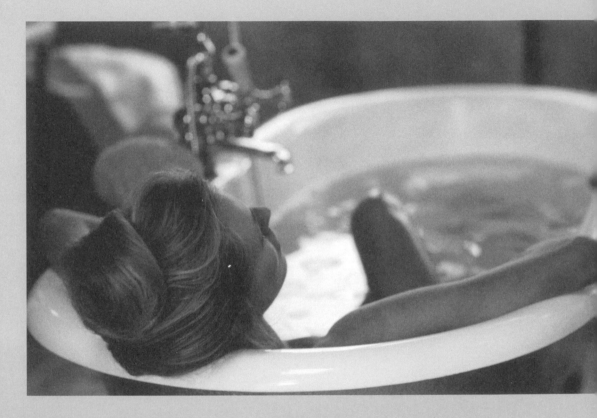

Relaxing in a deliciously fragrant bath scented with fresh herbs can help you wind down at the end of a hectic day and induce a restorative night's sleep.

External uses of herbs

You can also use herbs externally as many of their essential components are able to penetrate the skin.

Herbal baths

Pamper yourself in a long, warm herbal bath which will also have a medicinal effect. A few drops of essential oils can be added to the bath water just before you get in. The oils are carried on the steam and breathed in through the nose. Alternatively, you can fill a small muslin bag with a mixture of fresh aromatic herbs and hang it around the hot tap so that the water runs through the herbs as you fill the bath. If you have made a herbal infusion, you can pour it into your bath water.

Hand and foot baths have also been used for generations to treat a variety of problems. To make one of these, simply add a herbal

HERBAL REMEDIES

COMMON PROBLEM	RECOMMENDED HERB	METHOD OF APPLICATION
INFERTILITY CAUSED BY HORMONAL IMBALANCE	*Vitex agnus castus (chaste tree or hemp tree) • False unicorn root • Wild yam • Ginseng • Chinese angelica*	*Internally – in decoctions, infusions, or tincture form, either singly or in combination, three times daily*
ANAEMIA	*Comfrey leaves • Burdock leaves • Gentian • Yellow dock root • Raspberry leaves • Centaury • Hawthorn • Rosehips • Hops • Skullcap • Vervain*	*Internally – make a decoction or an infusion, either singly or in combination, and drink three times daily*
BACKACHE	*Ginger • Cinnamon • Lavender • Rosemary • Marshmallow • Couch grass rhizomes • Horsetail • Corn silk • Buchu • Cone flower • Raspberry leaves*	*Internally – make an infusion or decoction, either singly or in combination, and drink a lukewarm or cold cup every 20 minutes*
CONSTIPATION	*Burdock • Yellow dock root • Fennel • Raspberry leaves • Dandelion root • Linseed • Psyllium seeds*	*Internally – make an infusion or decoction and drink up to three times daily, or take one teaspoon of tincture*
CRAMP	*Horsetail • Comfrey leaf • Nettles • Kelp • Meadowsweet • Wild oats • Cramp bark • Hawthorn leaves, flowers and berries • Ginger*	*Internally – make an infusion or decoction, either singly or in combination, and drink a cupful three times daily*
HEARTBURN	*• Meadowsweet • Peppermint • Lemon balm*	*Internally – make an infusion or decoction and slowly sip at least two cupfuls throughout the day*

(continued)

COMMON PROBLEM	RECOMMENDED HERB	METHOD OF APPLICATION
HIGH BLOOD PRESSURE	*Hawthorn flowers, leaves and berries • Lime flowers • Passion flower • Cramp bark • Yarrow*	*Internally – take a cupful of an infusion or decoction, or take one teaspoon of tincture in a little water, three times daily.*
FLUID RETENTION	*Corn silk • Pellitory of the wall • Horsetail • Dandelion leaves • Couch grass rhizomes • Cleavers • Plantain*	*Internally – take a cupful of an infusion or decoction three times daily*
INSOMNIA	*Skullcap • Passionflower • Catnip • Valerian • Vervain • Chamomile • Lavender • Lemon balm • Raspberry leaves • Lime flower*	*Internally – take a cupful of an infusion or decoction, either singly or in combination, or take 1–2 teaspoons of tincture at night*
THRUSH	*Marigold • Rosemary • Oregano • Thyme • Fennel seed • Chamomile • American cranesbill • Beth root • Cone flower • Cleavers • Wild indigo*	*Externally – make an infusion or tincture and hold herb-soaked pads to the vulva, or add to sitz bath (hot steam cabinet in which you sit), or bathe the affected area frequently with it*

infusion, essential oils, or fresh or dried herbs to a bowl of warm water. Immerse your feet in the water for about 8 minutes in the morning, and your hands for the same length of time in the evening. Both the hands and feet are especially sensitive parts of the body, through which the medicinal qualities of the plants are able to pass. They can then be absorbed into the bloodstream.

Ointments and creams

These are suitable for certain conditions, such as varicose veins and haemorrhoids, and to prevent stretchmarks. They can be bought from herbal suppliers, or you can prepare them yourself at home very simply.

Soften 350g (12oz) of fresh or dried herbs in a mixture of pure olive oil and beeswax. You should use enough olive oil to cover the plant –

about 450ml (16 fl oz) – and 55g (2oz) of beeswax. If this is left on a low heat for a few hours in a bain-marie, the medicinal constituents of the plant will be taken up by the oil. Take the pan off the heat and pour the mixture into a muslin bag. Squeeze the oil and wax mixture through the muslin into a bowl and discard the herbs. The liquid mixture can then be poured into pots, and left to cool and solidify into an ointment.

Creams can be prepared simply by mixing a few drops of essential oil or herbal tincture into a jar of aqueous cream. You can get this from your local pharmacist.

Compresses

A clean cloth wrung out in a hot or cold herbal infusion or decoction can be applied repeatedly, if necessary, to affected areas. Alternatively, you can use water containing a few drops of an essential oil.

Poultices

These are another useful form of external administration, using the fresh or dried plant. The fresh herb needs to be bruised, and the dried herb needs to be powdered and mixed with water to form a paste. It is then applied to the affected part and bound with a light cotton bandage. This can be covered with clear film to avoid staining clothes. Poultices are usually applied hot, and can be kept warm using a hot-water bottle.

Herbs to be avoided

Most herbal remedies are generally safe during all stages of pregnancy. There are, however, certain herbs that should not be used pre-conceptually or during pregnancy as they can cause contraction of the uterus and could therefore threaten miscarriage:

Arbor vitae • autumn crocus • barberry • black cohosh • bloodroot • blue cohosh • broom • cotton root • feverfew • golden seal • greater celandine • juniper • life root • male fern • mistletoe • mugwort • nutmeg (in large quantities) • pennyroyal • poke root • rue • southernwood • tansy • thuja • wormwood

The consultation

At the first consultation, the medical herbalist will take a full case history, including details of your present condition and factors affecting your general health. He or she will want to know about your menstrual and reproductive history, any miscarriage, any previous illness, past drug therapy and inoculations and any reactions to them, allergies, any family tendencies to disease, stresses in your life, your general energy levels and emotional state, and your normal diet and lifestyle. The herbalist will also examine you.

The herbalist will prescribe plant remedies, as well as recommending changes in diet and lifestyle, including exercise, relaxation, and

REMEDIES FOR EMOTIONAL ISSUES

Bach flower remedies are available over the counter and may help with emotional upset.
Follow the labels for recommended dosage.

RECOMMENDED HERB	PARTICULAR PROBLEMS
LARCH	*Lack of confidence; fear of failure; not trying hard enough to succeed*
PINE	*Guilt; tendency to take the blame for other people's mistakes*
ELM	*Feeling overburdened by responsibility, which causes depression*
SWEET CHESTNUT	*Feeling of unbearable anguish; at end of tether*
STAR OF BETHLEHEM	*Great distress following some kind of shock, such as bad news*
WILLOW	*Bitterness or resentment about misfortune; the feeling that life is unjust*
OAK	*Refusal ever to give up, in spite of setbacks; struggling against all the odds*
CRAB APPLE	*Self-disgust; low self-esteem; the need to cleanse either mind or body*

referrals if necessary. Counselling is often very much part of the consultation.

Many herbal remedies are available over the counter in health food stores and pharmacies, and herbal medicine is one of the easiest of the natural therapies to use during your pregnancy. You can easily grow many of the medicinal herbs yourself, such as chamomile, thyme, rosemary, lavender, raspberry leaves, mint, wormwood, and feverfew. These can then be harvested and dried or used fresh and prepared as teas or tinctures.

Homeopathy

Homeopathy is a gentle form of medicine, which can be useful pre-conceptually and in pregnancy and labour. It is a holistic therapy, which works on both an emotional and a physical level by encouraging the body to heal itself.

The origins of homeopathy go back to 1910, when a German physician, Samuel Hahnemann, devised a new system of medicine as an alternative to the harsh conventional practices of the day, such as bloodletting and purging. His idea was to base his new system on gentle ways of helping the body to heal itself.

Hahnemann was inspired by the discovery that there was a herbal remedy for malaria which could also provoke the symptoms of the disease it was intended to treat. This discovery revived an ancient medical principle, first put forward by Hippocrates in the 5th century BC, that "like cures like". Hahnemann believed that small doses were better than large ones and devised a system of diluting doses to the maximum degree.

Homeopathy is a holistic therapy, which concentrates on the whole person – addressing their mental, emotional, spiritual, and physical aspects – and not just on the specific ailment that is being presented. It is a complex system of medicine, which aims to restore the body's natural balance and to strengthen its resistance to disease.

Before and during pregnancy

Homeopathic remedies are made from naturally occurring substances, such as plants, minerals and, in some cases, animals. Remedies are perfectly safe to take in pregnancy and, if used correctly, do not have any side-effects.

The ideal time to have homeopathic treatment is before conception, when both partners should be treated. This treatment raises your level of health and increases your chances of conception, as well as preparing you for a healthy pregnancy.

Both pre-conceptually and throughout the pregnancy, you can benefit from good "constitutional" treatment, which aims to treat your general constitution rather than any specific condition or ailment. Constitutional treatment will help keep you and your baby healthy throughout your pregnancy.

One of homeopathy's great strengths is that it can help to eradicate familial tendencies to illness. For example, if you or your partner – or perhaps both of you – suffers from eczema, your child stands a higher than average chance

115

of suffering from it, too. Treatment based on knowledge of your and your partner's combined health, and that of both your families, can deeply affect the health of your unborn child and lessen the possibility of inherited disorders.

Homeopathy can be useful at all stages of pregnancy, and many pregnant women choose to visit their homeopath once a month. It can be used to cure morning sickness and cramps, prevent constipation, and help with labour, as well as assisting in healing after birth. It relieves post-natal depression and homeopathy has saved many mothers with engorged breasts from abandoning the struggle to breastfeed.

The consultation

The aim of the homeopathic consultation is, first of all, to find out what kind of person you are. The homeopath will obviously want to know about your physical discomforts but he or she will also need to know how they affect you emotionally – whether they make you feel weepy or irritable, say – which will determine which remedy would be best for you.

The homeopath will ask you myriad questions about yourself, some of which may seem strange. You may be asked, for example, about your likes and dislikes in food, drink, and climate, whether you like company or prefer to be alone, whether you sweat, what anxieties or fears you have, and how well or badly you sleep. The answers to all these questions will help the

practitioner build up a detailed picture of you, which, in turn, will be matched to a remedy.

The homeopath may prescribe pulsatilla for women with no periods or irregular periods. Men may be treated with lycopodium, argentum nitricum, and selenium metallicum, but treatment will be on an individual basis.

Two consultations may be enough, but it is not uncommon for follow-up visits to be necessary – and possibly for quite some time if the condition is a chronic one. It is best to be treated professionally but, on occasions, self-prescribing may be helpful.

Homeopathic remedies

Remedies come in different strengths, or potencies. Those usually available from health food stores and pharmacies are the 6 and 30

TAKING REMEDIES

Tip the tablet on to your palm and put it under your tongue to dissolve. Do this at least 15 minutes before or after eating or drinking. Certain substances can stop remedies working. These include:

mint in all its forms, including toothpaste (fennel toothpaste, available in health food shops, is a good alternative) • tea • sweets • chewing gum • coffee • menthol • camphor • eucalyptus

potencies. The higher the number, the greater the dilution of the remedy and, according to Hahnemann's system, the greater its strength.

The 6 potency can be repeated hourly for up to six doses and the 30 potency can be repeated three-hourly for up to six doses. As soon as you start to feel any change, either physical or emotional, stop taking the remedy. This may be after just one dose, or it may be after several. The reaction shows that the healing process has been triggered and will continue of its own accord. If you continue taking the remedy, the body will become over-stimulated and your symptoms may intensify. If, however, there has been no change after six doses, you should seek professional help, as you may not have chosen the correct remedy.

Sometimes remedies can aggravate your symptoms temporarily. If this happens, stop taking the tablets and wait. After this initial intensification of symptoms, you should begin to feel better.

Both you and your partner may attend a homeopathic consultation in order to raise your general levels of health. This may work to increase your chances of conception as well as boosting all the systems of the body to prepare you for pregnancy.

Homeopathic remedies are made from naturally occurring substances such as plants and minerals.

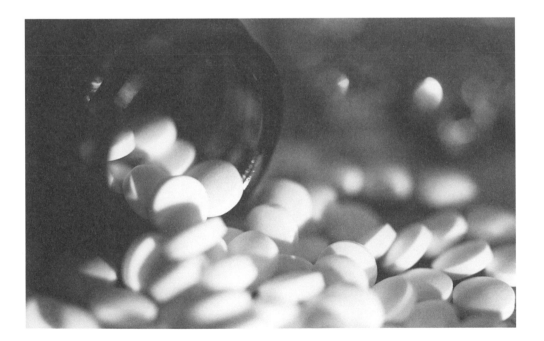

When
conception
is delayed

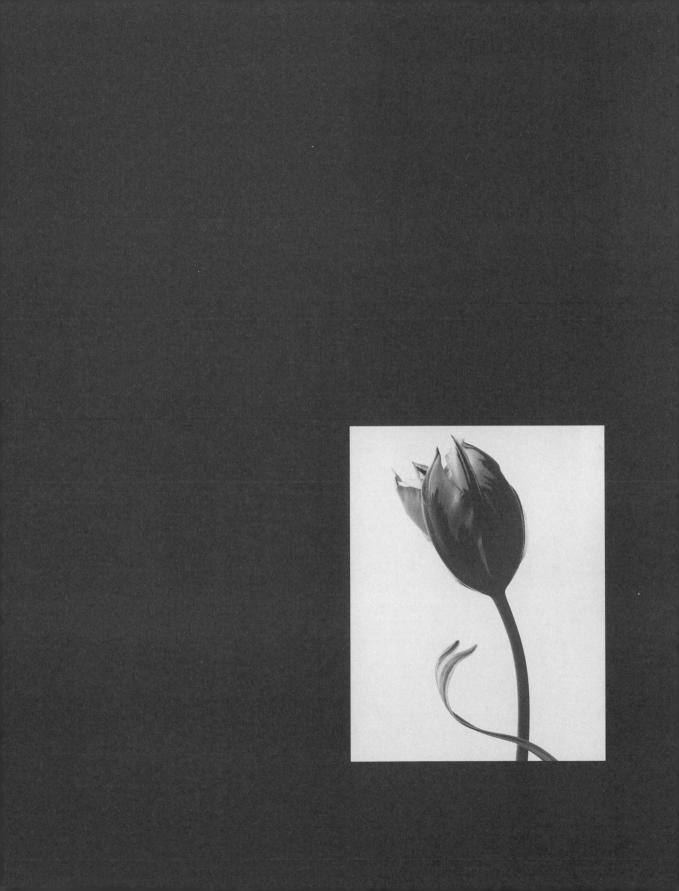

Understanding your feelings

Some people seem to be able to accept delays and difficulties in becoming pregnant with calm and equanimity, but others find the idea of being unable to fulfil this function deeply distressing and disappointing. As time goes by, some couples experience a roller-coaster of emotions, ranging from disbelief, despair, despondency, anger, frustration, and guilt, to a feeling of emptiness, a lack of fulfilment, and a sense of failure.

The woman's confidence may take a battering, her self-esteem may dip, and she may feel as if she is in an emotional turmoil, with each passing month bringing repeated disappointment. Waiting to discover whether or not she is going to have a period may start to dominate the other areas of her life, and she may find herself constantly waiting for the right time – her fertile period – and then grieving when pregnancy doesn't occur.

She may also feel astonished and angry that pregnancy does not happen easily and spontaneously, particularly if she has spent years using various contraceptive methods in order not to become pregnant at the wrong time or with the wrong partner.

She may now feel an acute sense of failure. This feeling can be especially strong if her partner has already had a child by a former partner. She may start to ask herself: "Why can't I do this?". However, it is perfectly possible for a

The most important thing for couples in this situation to remember is that they should never give up hope. What is known as unexplained infertility can just as easily, in time, give way to unexplained fertility.

man to father a child earlier in his life and subsequently to produce a low sperm count as he gets older – so even in these cases medical investigation of the man is always advisable in cases of delayed conception.

The woman may start to feel, if she believes that the delay in becoming pregnant is somehow her "fault", that she is letting her partner down, that her partner may become so disappointed that he will start to look outside the partnership. She may also feel guilty, particularly if she has had a termination of pregnancy in the past. Similarly, if she has had numerous partners, she may wonder if promiscuity or past infections have anything to do with her not getting pregnant.

She may start to feel angry and guilty that she is having to calculate her fertile period and concentrate on making love only on those days. Her partner, on the other hand, may come to regret the lack of spontaneity in their lovemaking and start to wonder if she wants a child more than she wants him.

These feelings are not uncommon but they are irrational: both partners should avoid apportioning blame or guilt, on themselves or on each other. Both partners in this distressing situation need a great deal of loving support, patience, and reassurance, both from one another and also from their friends and family members, if they are aware of the situation.

One couple in every seven will experience delays and difficulties in conception. Remember that it may easily take a year or more to become pregnant, even in couples where both partners have no fertility problems. Infertility is defined as the inability to become pregnant for more than one year of regular, unprotected sexual intercourse during the woman's fertile period.

Some couples do not become pregnant for two or more years, despite there being nothing

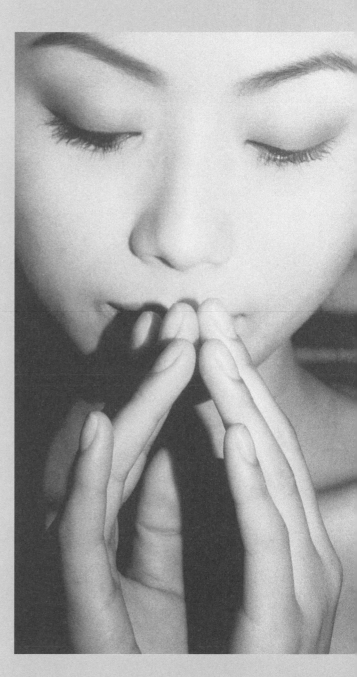

A woman who has difficulty in conceiving, or who suffers from repeated miscarriages, may become convinced that the fault lies with her and feel guilty that she is letting her partner down.

amiss with either partner. Every gynaecologist has had experience of hundreds of cases in which conception has been delayed, and then at last, for no obvious reason, the problem suddenly resolves itself and the woman becomes pregnant.

For example, a couple had been trying for ten years to become pregnant. They had all but accepted that their lives were going to be child-free. They did not want and could not afford expensive and intrusive medical assistance, and decided to accept the situation they found themselves in. However now, many years later, they have three gorgeous, healthy children – to their lasting surprise and joy. And that is just one case out of many thousands that have had a happy outcome.

Acceptance

In the meantime, it is important to recognize the damaging effect of repeated monthly disappointments on your partner and the impact of delayed conception on your other relationships, on your family, and on how you manage at work. It is vital to avoid damaging your relationship with your life partner for the sake of a need that may get out of control and develop into an obsession.

A truly good relationship is the most valuable gift in life and something that deeply enriches all the other areas of your life. There is a need to enjoy life as it is, as it is offered to you. One

cannot always be looking to the future, we all need to try to live in the present.

Of course, it is easy to feel irritable and jealous of friends and family who have young children, and to feel hopeless and helpless about your own continued childlessness. If your sister or sister-in-law becomes pregnant, this may present a very painful and uncomfortable hurdle to cross. It may prove difficult to forget your own situation and congratulate others on their good fortune.

It is easy to become swept up in a cycle of disbelief, anger, grief, guilt, and frustration. It is easy to feel angry at the sight of a young mother with one child in a pushchair, one walking by her side, and another on the way. Why, you may ask yourself, should you need help with the most natural event in the world?

All these feelings are very natural and completely understandable, but you need to regain a perspective on your life as a whole with your partner and rejoice in what you already have in your own life.

In cases of "accepted" infertility, it is sometimes just at the time when both partners have accepted that they will not have children, that the woman becomes pregnant. One couple underwent three years of infertility treatments, all to no avail. Within one year of accepting that their lives were to be with one another but not with children, the woman became pregnant and the couple now have four lovely daughters. There are many known cases, too, of couples who have adopted a child, only then for the woman to become pregnant within a year or two and give birth to a healthy child.

There may come a time during the long and painful wait for a pregnancy to become established when one considers medical assistance and intervention. This is a deeply personal choice and one that some couples may decide against. Others, however, will wish to take whatever steps are possible in order to have a child. (The options available are described in Knowing when to seek help, pages 132–41.)

The need for support

Part of the stress that is caused by difficulty with conceiving results from not knowing what the future will bring. In fact, the future is equally unpredictable for everyone, and an event that occurs tomorrow could change your life forever, but we need to feel in control of our lives. When you want a child and cannot conceive, you have a feeling of putting all your plans for the future on hold, which naturally contributes to a sense of emotional turmoil. Should I take that new job? Do I risk a house move and by so doing perhaps fail to conceive yet again? Why move at all if we are never going to need extra space? Does our new home need to be near good schools? Whose "fault" is it? Is it me? Is it my partner? Why is this happening to us?

The anguish and corrosive effect that delayed conception can have on all one's

relationships need to be acknowledged and understood, primarily by both partners, but also by other family members and friends, if they are to be sympathetic to the couple. Delayed conception, miscarriage, and infertility – and the very deep feelings that these situations provoke – have the potential for irretrievably damaging a relationship.

Miscarriage brings its own uniquely wounding sense of loss for both partners. The loss of a baby, however young, represents a bereavement. The loss of the child needs to be fully acknowledged and grieved for by both partners. The question of what might have been is all the more poignant and distressing in cases of miscarriage.

Recurrent or repeated miscarriage (three or more), presents an emotional and physical hurdle for both partners, the more so for the woman. Again, the situation may demand sustained support for both partners from their friends and relatives.

It is well known that a delay in becoming pregnant and giving birth to a healthy baby is a major cause of psychological and marital stress. For this reason, the rest of this chapter is devoted to a number of therapies that may help in alleviating stress and anxiety.

It is important that the two partners can still enjoy one another, can continue to enrich one another's lives, and can be able to give one another the support, reassurance, and love that each of them needs.

123

Relaxation techniques

The anxiety, frustration, and despair that may be experienced by couples who fail to conceive relatively quickly can be alleviated to some degree by taking a positive attitude to life. Relaxation techniques can help couples to cope with stress when conception is delayed.

Some of the complementary therapies can be used in the same way as exercise, both as specific treatment and as a general part of your lifestyle. You may already have your favourite therapy, for there are now many to choose from. The next few pages describe a selection of those therapies that are particularly suited for treating the conditions of sadness, despair, and anxiety, which are some of the feelings you may experience if it takes longer to become pregnant than you had anticipated.

The previous chapter looked at how therapies and techniques can be incorporated into your lifestyle, whether you are intending to become pregnant, are already pregnant, or are experiencing difficulty in conceiving. This chapter looks at more specific therapies for the relief of anxiety.

What is termed "unexplained" infertility accounts for a large proportion of cases of delayed conception. Therefore, the benefits of all the techniques shown on pages 86–117, together with those that follow, cannot be underestimated.

Visualization

With this therapy, you can choose to focus on positive images and the desired outcome to specific situations in which you find yourself. This allows you to cope with your problems and see your way through your despair. What you visualize may become reality.

Creating mental pictures to relieve despondency and to alleviate anxiety is a technique that has been used in many parts of the world for many years. It possesses tremendous potential for you, your partner, and your child-to-be.

The patient is encouraged to draw a picture in his or her mind that will boost positive feelings about his or her self-image, physical and mental health, and future life.

Visualization is a technique that was used by witch doctors in Africa and South America in early times and formed an important part of early oriental therapies. In the West, its history goes back to the civilization of ancient Greece, where it was considered to be a crucial factor in healing illness. In the 1920s, a lot of work was

124

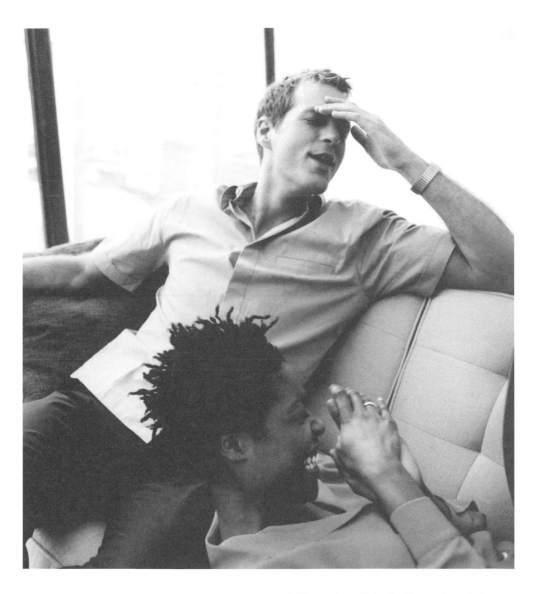

A host of recognized techniques are available amongst the complementary therapies to help you relax and reduce anxiety. On a less formal level, ordinary enjoyable activities that help you to look outside your immediate situation are important. Laughing is therapeutic, and even if you don't think you can face other people, time spent in the company of good, supportive friends will have a positive effect.

126

done on visualization therapy with cancer patients by a doctor called Carl Simonton, who practised radiotherapy in Texas.

Simonton was convinced that a person's reaction to disease played an important part in both its onset and its cure. He and his wife asked cancer patients to create mental pictures of their cancer cells being attacked and destroyed by healthy ones. They became convinced that patients who took part in this programme lived about twice as long as others and that, in some cases, the illness stopped spreading altogether.

The visualization therapist will listen to your detailed description of the problem. He or she will then encourage you to relax in a comfortable position. The therapist will tell you to imagine a scene that relates to your particular situation. It may be a real scene, which you remember from a painting, a film, or a photograph, or it may be an imaginary scene.

As you describe the scene you are visualizing, the therapist will encourage you to describe what you are feeling. If he or she thinks you should alter what you are visualizing in any way, you will be encouraged to do so.

Meditation

The ancient eastern art of achieving spiritual enlightenment can be used as a way of shedding the anxieties and stresses caused by delayed fertility.

VISUALIZATION TECHNIQUES

In general, it is most effective to be taught the technique of visualization by a specialist. After your consultation, you can practise the technique at home, following these steps:

- *Choose a time when you know that you will have a clear 30 minutes to yourself, without interruption; switch off the telephone*

- *Select a comfortable chair to sit in, or, in you prefer, lie down on your back on the floor*

- *Close your eyes*

- *Begin to imagine a scene that represents for you peace and tranquillity. It may be the open moors, or a seascape with waves calmly lapping at the edge of the beach, a silent mountain landscape or a beautiful garden. It may be a real place that you have visited, or an ideal landscape. What matters is that its message is quiet and relaxing*

- *Allow yourself to be drawn into your picture and exclude everything else in your life*

- *Now visualize the specific situation that you wish for and allow your mind the freedom to explore*

- *When you have finished, get up slowly*

(You can do this on a train or bus journey, just as well as at home.)

Meditation has been practised for centuries in India and much of Asia. It came to prominence in the West in the 1960s, when many people became interested in it as an alternative way of dealing with life's problems. In the 21st century it continues to have a huge following among the general public.

Meditation is regarded by its practitioners as the ultimate form of self-help, in which you calm both mind and body by controlling your powers of concentration.

Physical benefits that follow a period of meditation include lower blood pressure and a slower pulse rate and, if you practise it regularly, long-term benefits may also result, including better circulation, relief from frequent headaches, easier breathing, and a cure for persistent insomnia.

There are several different schools of thought on meditation. Each holds different views about the goal of meditation, and how best to do it. Probably the best-known is the method devised by the Maharishi Mahesh Yogi and his disciples, which is known as transcendental meditation (TM).

Many people find it impossible to begin meditating on their own and will benefit from being taught the initial techniques by an expert teacher. The preliminaries of meditation may include adopting a certain posture, which may be lying down on the floor or sitting upright in a position that you can maintain comfortably. You may be given a mantra – a sound or phrase that

MEDITATION TECHNIQUES

- *Lie on your back on the floor with the palms of your hands outstretched and facing upward. Place a cushion under your neck and make sure that you are comfortable*
- *Close your eyes*
- *Consciously relax every part of your body, one part at a time*
- *Concentrate on your feet and toes. Let them relax*
- *Now focus on your legs, concentrating on relaxing first your calves and then your knees and thighs*
- *Make sure that your spine is supple and relaxed, with your shoulders lying flat to the floor and as opened out as possible*
- *Let your arms go and relax your wrists and hands*
- *Concentrate on your breathing. Be aware of your abdominal muscles becoming more relaxed as your breathing deepens and slows. Let your mind float freely*
- *Experience your worries floating away out of your body, and allow your spirit to relax*
- *Remain like this for up to 20 minutes, without going to sleep*
- *Gradually bring your mind back to the present. Get up slowly when you are ready and stretch out your limbs, one by one, and then your back*

127

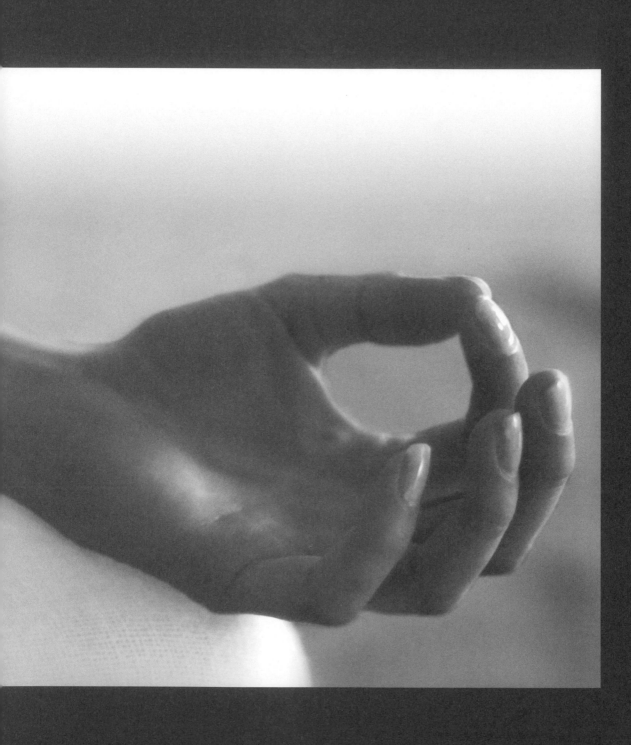

is repeated over and over again to calm your mind and silence the chatter of a busy mind.

It is best not to eat or drink for about half an hour before meditating. You need a warm, quiet room, where you will not be disturbed. You may begin by concentrating on slow, deep breathing, which will help empty your mind of troublesome thoughts. When your breathing becomes completely automatic, unwanted thoughts may stray into your head and you may need to transfer your concentration from your breath to a conscious effort to relax each part of your body in turn.

Once you've learned how to meditate, you will be able to do it on your own at home. As you become better at it, you will probably find that you can turn on a meditative state virtually anywhere and at any time – not just at home but also on the bus, on the train, between household chores, and in your lunch break.

Hypnotherapy

Inducing an altered state of consciousness, somewhere between being awake and being asleep, can have a surprisingly powerful effect on your health. A hypnotherapist uses a

Meditating on a regular basis is a satisfying way to gain deep relaxation. Your mind quietens and your thoughts cease to be a burden and a distraction. Instead, the mind becomes a tool for paying full attention to the present moment. The physical benefits of meditation include lower blood pressure, better sleep patterns and recovery from fatigue.

patient's altered state of consciousness to bring about changes, either physical or mental, in that patient. These can include a range of positive changes, such as healing disorder and illness, causing the patient to relax, and preventing or easing pain.

Pain relief was one of the earliest uses of hypnosis. By the 1820s, the public was familiar with the power of hypnotism to relieve pain, though many doctors remained sceptical. In the mid- to late 19th century, some surgeons took to using hypnotherapy for some of their patients undergoing operations. In spite of its obvious success in the field of pain relief, hypnotherapy went into a decline by the end of the 19th century. This was largely as a result of the arrival of quick and easy anaesthetics, such as ether and chloroform.

It is only in the last 60 years or so that hypnotherapy has been revived. Therapists see the half-way state between wakefulness and sleep as a state of limbo, in which mind and body reach a calmness and equilibrium that are conducive to healing. Hypnotherapy has been used successfully in the treatment of headaches, digestive problems, fertility disorders, skin disorders, asthma, insomnia, phobias, and many other conditions associated with stress and anxiety. Hypnosis can also be used to cure addictions such as smoking, drugs, and alcohol.

At your first session, the therapist will take a detailed case history and will also discuss how

129

130

you see your current problem. He or she will probably not hypnotize you at the first meeting, though they may test to see whether you are susceptible to hypnosis. Most people are susceptible, but a few people are not.

At the next session, you will sit or lie down and the therapist will hypnotize you. This is usually done by talking to you calmly, slowly, and quietly, and by suggesting that your eyelids are beginning to feel heavy and you are feeling sleepy. Sometimes the therapist will get you to focus your eyes on a particular object, which will increase your desire to shut your eyes. This all feels quite pleasant and you will probably feel as though you are dozing off.

It is while you are in this state that the therapist can get you to think about the future in as positive a way as possible. They can suggest that you look at problems from a new perspective, or they can instil a new resolve to deal with a particular problem.

A hypnotherapist will usually teach a patient to carry out self-hypnosis at home. Some therapists will also give their patient a tape recording, which will provide the right trigger for entering a trance-like state.

Talking cures

Talking to a friend when you are depressed and in distress can be of inestimable value. Talking things over with a friend can itself be described as supportive psychotherapy. Some forms of psychotherapy are similar to this, though the therapist – unlike the friend – knows that the importance of talking is that it gives you the opportunity to understand your situation. He or she will not, and is not expected to, tell you what you should do.

One common feature of all psychotherapies is the therapist's belief that they will be able to help modify their client's own feelings and views about themselves. A second common feature is that the therapist is not there to find answers to your problems. They allow you to find your own answers through the technique of exploratory discussion. By developing your own strategies, you will develop in maturity and inner strength, thus forming the foundations for managing your life in the future.

The following therapies are all available through your family doctor:

Supportive psychotherapy

In essence, this involves sharing your perceived problems with a warm and sympathetic ear. Many different health professionals are trained to offer supportive psychotherapy, including doctors, specialist nurses, counsellors, psychologists, and health visitors.

Cognitive therapy

This, together with interpersonal therapy, is at the cutting edge of the psychotherapies practised at the start of the 21st century.

Cognition describes the mental activities of thinking, memory, and perception. Cognitive therapy may be defined as help with how you view events and situations in life. According to this therapy, the way in which you think determines how you feel, and it is believed that if you modify your automatic reactions and thoughts, your feelings and mood will subsequently be altered.

The aim is to identify and challenge negative and pessimistic thought patterns that have become entrenched, with a view to developing new, more realistic, and more objective thoughts. These new thoughts will by definition be more optimistic, so that your mood will be improved and despondency will start to lift.

The sufferer is encouraged to keep a diary to record moods, thoughts, and activities, to challenge stereotypical behaviour, to set targets, to carry out self-help tasks as homework, and to instigate a system of rewards for each small positive step.

Cognitive therapy is especially suitable for problems associated with low self-esteem and for patterns of destructive behaviour, such as anger and heavy drinking.

Interpersonal therapy

This is aimed at improving personal relationships. It is based on the view that the crucial factor in despair is the sufferer's social network or interpersonal relationships. These are determined to some extent by life events and by parental relationships. There may be a failure to achieve a harmonious relationship with one's parents despite many attempts, with the experience of being told repeatedly that one is stupid, naughty, unlovable, or incompetent. The loss of a parent while still a child can be very damaging psychologically.

Interpersonal therapy explores grief and loss reactions, conflicts with friends, family, and colleagues, social skills, and the problems of adjustment to major life events (such as bereavement, infertility, or loss of job) with a view to modifying the sufferer's perceptions.

Marital therapy

Counselling for relationship and marital problems can prove helpful as it affords both parties the opportunity to air their grievances in the presence of an objective third party in an atmosphere that is constructive rather than destructive. Solutions and compromises may be achieved. See Finding help on pages 154–5.

Group therapy

A group of people, united by the similarity of their problems, are given psychotherapy together. This can prove helpful in that it shows each sufferer that they are not alone. Similarly, each member can contribute to the progress and well-being of the rest of the group by posing questions, offering constructive criticism, and by appraisal and encouragement. See Finding help on pages 154–5.

131

Knowing
when to seek
help

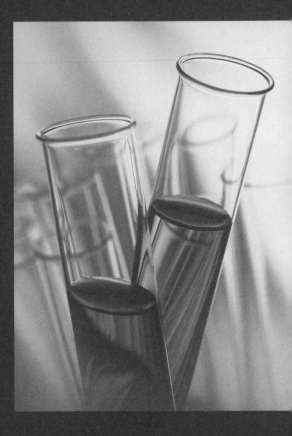

Professional help

Infertility is defined as more than one year of regular unprotected sexual intercourse without pregnancy occurring. At this point, it is wise to seek professional help, through your own doctor, in the form of fertility investigation and possible treatment at the nearest hospital-assisted conception unit.

Infertility today does not necessarily mean that you will not have children. There is no need to resign yourself to the distress caused by delay or inability to conceive if you are prepared to contemplate medical intervention. Before this stage is reached, investigation of both partners may reveal a problem that can be resolved, leading to spontaneous conception.

If you have never been pregnant, the problem is defined as primary infertility. If you have been pregnant before (whether or not the pregnancy was successful), but are now experiencing delay in conceiving, it is termed secondary infertility. You should also seek an early appointment with a hospital consultant gynaecologist if you have suffered more than three miscarriages.

fertility treatments and for assisted fertility treatments are not that high. For example, there is a 10 per cent chance of conception each month, at best, after any fertility surgery.

However, the picture is not all gloomy. There are successes, and many couples who have sought professional help have been fortunate enough to conceive and have a child. In some cases, they have had more than one child. It should be remembered, however, that infertility treatments may be – and usually are – time-consuming, often drawn out over a long period of time (sometimes years), expensive, and intrusive. It also needs to be borne in mind, when embarking on such a course, that many people can find fertility investigations and treatments painful and distressing.

The success rate

Much has been written in the media about miracle developments in fertility. Much of it is, unfortunately, misleading, in that miracle cures do not exist and the success rates for routine

General health

Once you decide to seek professional help, the fertility specialists will check out your general health and lifestyle before commencing with routine fertility treatments.

134

In the case of the man, the specialist will probably advise:

- losing excess weight
- stopping smoking (which, if continued, may render any fertility treatment useless)
- reducing alcohol intake to a minimum
- abstaining from caffeine
- abstaining from drugs – cannabis and cocaine, for example, both adversely affect sperm quality and quantity
- avoiding excessive exercise
- monitoring the temperature of the testicles (if they are too hot, conception may not take place)
- reducing stress
- avoiding occupations that carry a greater risk to fertility: in pneumatic drill operators, for instance, excessive vibration can affect sperm production; and in occupational car drivers the testicles may become too hot to produce sperm
- coming off medication that may interfere with sperm production, unless it is vital that the medication is continued

It should be noted that it takes some 70 days for the man to make sperm and it is therefore important that the man has complied with all these lifestyle pointers for some four months before semen analysis is carried out.

In the case of the woman, the specialist will probably advise:

- losing excess weight
- stopping smoking
- abstaining from alcohol completely for the time being
- abstaining from drugs
- following a healthy diet
- taking regular exercise
- being sure to get enough good-quality, regular sleep
- setting time aside for relaxation at least every other day

The woman's menstrual cycle and ovulatory cycle will be investigated, to check her hormone levels of oestrogen, progesterone, luteinizing hormone, and follicle stimulating hormone (see Understanding your fertility, pages 12–43) and to check her general health, as well as looking at the health of her reproductive system.

Routine fertility treatments

It is essential to have all the appropriate routine fertility treatments that are possible before resorting to any of the high-tech, high-profile assisted conception treatments now available.

Tests are necessary to establish that the woman is producing eggs, that the man is producing sufficient numbers of sperm, that the sperm are of adequate quality, and that the sperm are able to meet the eggs. The results of these tests will dictate which of the following techniques are appropriate.

135

> **ROUTINE FERTILITY TREATMENTS**
>
> *These may include:*
>
> * *Fertility medication – such as clomiphene, which stimulates ovulation, and other drugs in certain cases*
> * *Surgery or microsurgery, either to ovaries or Fallopian tubes*
> * *Laparoscopic surgery*
> * *Laser surgery*

Artificial insemination

AIH (artificial insemination by the husband), involves inseminating the woman with her partner's sperm, in hospital, by means of a syringe at the time she is ovulating.

This method is appropriate for couples in which the woman's body makes antibodies to her partner's sperm, destroying them before they reach the egg. It is also useful for couples who experience sexual difficulties such as vaginismus or male impotence, and for unexplained infertility.

Donor insemination

DI (donor insemination) involves inseminating the woman with an unidentified donor's sperm, in hospital, by means of a syringe when she is ovulating. This method is appropriate for cases when the male partner is impotent or has defective sperm.

Intrauterine insemination

IUI involves the introduction of sperm directly into the woman's uterus, in hospital, through the vagina and cervix. The sperm are treated first and the woman may be given fertility drugs to stimulate the ovaries to help her produce more than one egg at the time of ovulation. If the sperm are normal or nearly normal, the success rate is higher than that of IVF.

This measure enhances the chances of conception by artificial insemination and is sometimes used in cases of male impotence or other sexual difficulty, or unexplained infertility, in place of ICSI (see page 138).

In vitro fertilization

So-called test-tube babies are conceived in a procedure that fertilizes the woman's eggs with her husband's sperm outside her body. The first successful in vitro fertilization (IVF) treatment

> **WHAT ARE THE OPTIONS FOR ASSISTED FERTILITY?**
>
> *Once a diagnosis has been made of the reasons for a couple's infertility, and medical intervention is found to be necessary, there is a range of options to choose from. All the various options fall into one of two groups: artificial insemination and the various methods of assisted conception.*

occurred in 1978 and resulted in what became known as the first test-tube baby. For this reason it is often known as the test-tube method, although, in fact, the egg is fertilized in a dish and the resulting embryo transferred into the woman's uterus.

As the first step in the procedure, the woman's ovaries are stimulated with drugs to produce eggs. These are collected and mixed with sperm. Once fertilized, the eggs are replaced in the woman's uterus in hospital. This technique can be used in cases of poor quality sperm, if the woman's body is making antibodies to the sperm, for unexplained infertility, blocked or scarred Fallopian tubes, or irregular ovulation.

The same technique is used as a test of the partner's sperm: if the egg becomes fertilized in a dish, it proves that the sperm is effective and makes further analysis of sperm unnecessary.

When IVF is to be carried out, the woman's ovaries are usually stimulated by fertility drugs. She is carefully monitored while taking these to measure the growth of ovarian follicles, to avoid the risk of hyperstimulation of the ovaries, and to reduce side-effects.

The eggs are usually collected under local anaesthetic, with additional sedation. They are removed using a small needle passed through the wall of the upper vagina (sometimes through a laparoscope), without the need for a general anaesthetic.

Provided that both eggs and sperm are healthy, approximately 60 per cent of the eggs will be fertilized. Two days after the eggs have been obtained, up to three embryos can be transferred directly into the uterine cavity. If the embryo attaches to the lining of the uterus, in the process known as implantation, pregnancy is the result.

The success rate for IVF varies considerably. When two embryos are transferred to the woman's uterus, there is generally a one in four chance of pregnancy. Of the 25 per cent of couples who succeed in achieving pregnancy with this method, some go on to have a child. What is known as the "take home" baby success rate for IVF is 14 per cent.

Gamete intra-Fallopian transfer

Women who have no problem with their Fallopian tubes can be offered this technique, which is a variation of in vitro fertilization. The eggs and sperm are collected as in IVF and placed together in the Fallopian tube, in hospital, and left to fertilize themselves. Doctors simply examine the eggs, usually selecting no more than three, and add sperm before replacing them both in the Fallopian tube. This is done by laparoscopy, which involves having an anaesthetic.

The woman must have healthy Fallopian tubes for GIFT to be used and to be successful. The "take home" baby success rate for this method can be as high as 26 per cent.

Zygote intra-Fallopian transfer

This is a combination of IVF and gamete intra-Fallopian transfer. The woman's eggs are collected in the same way as in IVF and the eggs are mixed with sperm in a test tube. Once fertilization has taken place, the fused egg and sperm is placed in the Fallopian tube by laparoscopy, and not in the uterus as in IVF. This technique is used when GIFT either has not worked or is considered unlikely to work because fertilization between egg and sperm has not happened naturally.

The woman's Fallopian tubes must be healthy and functioning in order for this method to be used and to be successful.

Pro nuclear stage embryo transfer

This is the same as the IVF procedure except that the fertilized eggs are placed in the Fallopian tube, in hospital, using a laparoscope rather than being introduced into the uterus through the vagina and cervix. The woman's Fallopian tubes must be healthy for this technique to be used.

Intra-cytoplasmic sperm injection

In this procedure, a single sperm is directly injected into an egg, in laboratory conditions. The egg will previously have been retrieved from the woman's ovary in the same way as it is for the IVF procedure.

This technique is especially suitable for couples in whom the sperm is of poor quality and quantity, and is therefore unable to fertilize an egg using IVF. Following the procedure, the embryos are placed into the uterus in the same way as in the IVF procedure.

Egg donation

This is the only technique available for women who are not producing eggs. Otherwise, the only alternatives are surrogacy or adoption.

The procedure involves another woman donating her egg or eggs to the couple. The eggs are then fertilized in a laboratory dish by the male partner's sperm. The resulting embryo is placed in the female partner's uterus and she is given hormonal drugs in order to maintain the pregnancy.

Women who may consider this option are those unable to produce eggs of their own, women who have inherited a genetic disease and who might pass on the disorder to their children, women over the age of 35 who have already tried IVF and for whom it has been unsuccessful, and women who have experienced a premature menopause.

Egg donation is a highly complex procedure, requiring the same drug treatment and monitoring before egg collection as IVF or GIFT.

Egg donors are usually young women who have already had their own children. Because of the high level of commitment required, the donor may be a relative or close friend of the couple.

Once the eggs are collected from the donor, they are fertilized with sperm from the recipient's partner. Up to three embryos are then transferred to the uterus. The success rate for this method is good but it is limited by a shortage of donors.

Surrogacy

A woman who has found that she is unable to carry a baby to term, or who is unable to conceive in any medically assisted way, may

A variety of procedures involve the fertilization of the egg outside the woman's body, in a laboratory dish, known as in vitro fertilization. This may involve simply mixing eggs with sperm, but it is also possible to inject a single sperm directly into an egg.

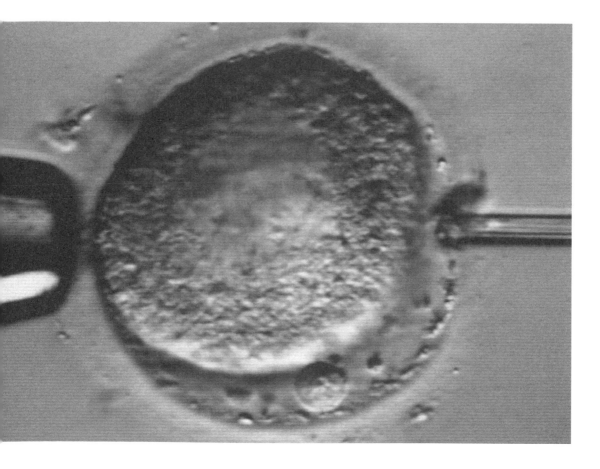

139

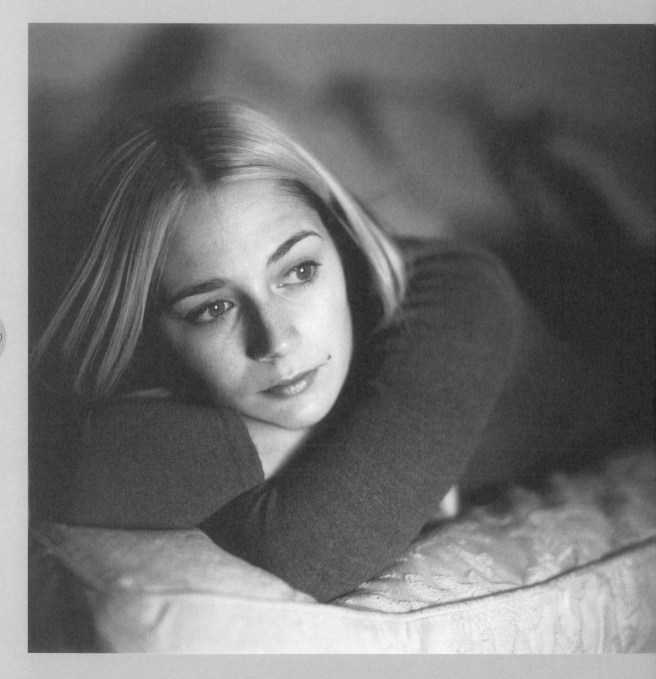

consider having another woman carry her own fertilized egg to full term and give birth to the baby on her behalf. In some cases, the surrogate mother conceives using the husband's sperm and her own egg, and then hands over the baby at birth.

Surrogacy is an emotionally and legally complex solution to infertility. A surrogate mother may form such a strong bond with the unborn child during the nine months of her pregnancy that she finds herself unable to give it up at birth. If this happens, much heartache will be caused to all the participants. Alternatively, a couple may leave themselves vulnerable to a dishonest surrogate mother who takes financial compensation but has no intention from the outset of handing over the baby when it is born. Even a successful surrogacy raises the problem of what to tell the child about his or her origins.

Apart from the emotional complexities, surrogacy is an extreme choice that is riddled with legal problems and complex regulations. It requires all parties to the arrangement to conform with the law, and to be fully aware and in written agreement about each aspect of the transaction. Payment for surrogacy is illegal in some countries, including the UK.

Whichever treatment you choose to undergo involves a high degree of commitment by both partners. You need to think carefully and realistically about the chances of success, and not to lose sight of all the positive aspects of your life, with or without a child.

Adoption

Adopting a child is the alternative for couples who either have not achieved success with the fertility treatments that have been offered to them, or who decide that they would prefer to adopt as a positive choice.

The legal situation surrounding adoption is much clearer than that of surrogacy, although upper age limits may apply, which may be a problem after a long period of infertility

Acceptance

Some couples may decide to go ahead with fertility treatments, while others may decline. Couples who are undergoing fertility investigations and treatments should always consider counselling as an extra means of emotional support. Similarly, couples who decide not to pursue fertility treatments may also wish to receive counselling, again as an extra source of support as they come to terms with their decision.

A surprising number of couples find that, within a few years of accepting infertility, to their great surprise and happiness, the woman becomes pregnant. As explained earlier in this book, unexplained infertility may sometimes, inexplicably, give way to unexplained fertility.

Whatever happens, the couple who accept infertility need to remember to rejoice in what they have together – to value one another and to live for the here and now.

141

Testing for pregnancy

Taking a pregnancy test

This may be the moment you have both longed for: you have missed a period, or possibly two successive periods, and you are about to take a pregnancy test. You are filled with feelings of anticipation and hope for the future.

For couples who have suffered the strains of delayed or difficult conception, this could be one of the great turning points of their lives.

You can take a pregnancy test just after you have missed a period. Tests taken any earlier than this can give false negative results and, rarely, false positive ones. You can arrange to have a pregnancy test done by your doctor, by a hospital, by a chemist, or by a family planning clinic. Alternatively, you can buy an over-the-counter pregnancy testing kit and do it yourself.

How pregnancy tests work

Pregnancy tests work by detecting and measuring the amount of one of the pregnancy hormones, human chorionic gonadotrophin (HCG), which is produced in the woman's bloodstream. The amount doubles every two or three days in the first six weeks of pregnancy.

Most pregnancy tests suggest that you use an early morning urine sample. This is because HCG is present in the bladder in its greatest concentrations first thing in the morning. In most tests, a urine sample is mixed with an anti-HCG substance. If the woman is pregnant, the urine will contain HCG, which will neutralize the anti-HCG. The mixture is then added to a suspension of particles coated with HCG. If she is pregnant, there will be no reaction because the anti-HCG has been neutralized. If she is not pregnant, the particles are agglutinated (they clump together) by the non-neutralized anti-HCG. Some of the more recent tests are based on colour changes. This is seen as a blue line in the window of a testing strip.

HOW RELIABLE ARE PREGNANCY TESTS?

If carried out by a doctor or chemist, these tests are pretty reliable. With home pregnancy testing kits, the following can affect the reliability of the test:

doing the test wrongly • doing it correctly but reading the result incorrectly • doing the test correctly and reading the result correctly, but the reactive substance fails to function properly

144

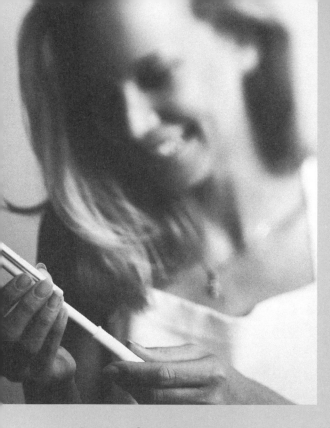

You may have waited years before taking a pregnancy test. If the first test is negative, repeat it a few days later when HCG levels will have increased.

A positive result

If the result is positive, you should see your doctor a couple of weeks later – bringing you to about eight weeks of pregnancy. The obstetrician may conduct an internal examination to confirm your pregnancy, although this is now less commonly done than previously. This involves inserting two fingers into your vagina and palpating your abdomen with the other hand, to detect a softening of the genital organs and the increase in size of the uterus.

Nowadays, it is more likely the pregnancy will be confirmed by ultrasound scan. If you are not overweight, a scan through the abdominal wall will show a heartbeat at seven weeks. Earlier, or if you are overweight, a scan through the vagina may be necessary. This does not increase the chance of miscarriage or damage the baby in any way. The alternative is to wait one more week for an abdominal scan.

If you are having slight vaginal bleeding and pelvic discomfort, a vaginal scan may be recommended to exclude ectopic pregnancy. This is important because an ectopic pregnancy that ruptures can be fatal. Tubal damage causing infertility may cause ectopic pregnancy. If you have had a previous ectopic pregnancy, this increases the chance of another one. Investigations must be undertaken to exclude it.

145

A negative result

If the first test is negative, repeat the test a few days later, by which time the level of HCG (if you are pregnant) will have increased. If the second result is negative, you are probably not pregnant.

This can be a bitter blow for a couple who are eager to have a child. It is important for them to work together to resolve this setback, and not let it cause a rift. Most importantly, neither partner should blame the other in any way. This is a shared enterprise and the ups and downs need to be shared likewise.

Should this turn out to be more than a minor setback and should infertility prove to be a real problem, the couple can talk to their doctor and discuss the next steps, as there is much that can be done to help them (see Knowing when to seek help, page 132).

Early signs and symptoms

There are some women who claim that they can tell that they are pregnant virtually from day one. They don't feel they need to wait for any symptoms – they just "know". Some people believe that this is something to do with the first secretions of the hormones of pregnancy. However, many others need something a little more tangible to prove that they are really pregnant – see pregnancy testing on page 144.

For most women, some or all of the following outward signs and symptoms are useful indicators that they are pregnant, and some of them may be experienced during the very first weeks after conception.

Tiredness

The first sign that you notice may be nothing more than tiredness. Some women feel energized at the beginning of pregnancy, but most women feel terribly tired in a strange way that they have not experienced before.

They may find that they become so tired by the middle of the afternoon, that they just have to stop whatever it is they are doing and wait for a feeling of tremendous lethargy to pass. Some women even find themselves dropping off to sleep in the middle of the day, even though they got out of bed only a few hours earlier after a perfectly normal night's sleep.

Missed period

The first definite sign of pregnancy is a missed period, which is known as amenorrhoea. While pregnancy is the most common cause of amenorrhoea, it is not the only one. You must not, therefore, automatically assume that you are pregnant, although, as you are trying to get pregnant, it is probably the most likely reason.

Morning sickness

Many women suffer from morning sickness, which is caused partly by an increased level of hormones circulating in the blood. The sudden rush of hormones can irritate the lining of the stomach, which manifests itself as nausea.

Morning sickness does often happen in the morning, but it can also happen at other times of the day. Indeed, some women are unlucky enough to feel sick for whole days at a time during the first few weeks. It can happen from

146

about week six and rarely lasts for longer than the first 15 weeks of pregnancy. Some women continue to experience nausea and sickness throughout pregnancy, but this is rare.

Urination

Another common early symptom is an increased frequency of urination, known as micturition. You may notice this as early as one week after conception. It is caused partly by the swelling uterus pressing on the bladder, which lies very close to the uterus, and partly because of the alterations in muscle tone due to hormonal changes. It tends to occur in the first eight to nine weeks of pregnancy. After this time, the uterus, containing the fetus, moves upwards, and the pressure on the bladder is thus relieved to some extent.

Some women, however, find that they need to pass water constantly throughout pregnancy. It is also not uncommon to be somewhat incontinent, so that when you laugh or cough, you involuntarily pass a little water. If this happens to you, wear well-fitting briefs and a light sanitary pad or panty liner.

Tender breasts

You may notice soreness and tingling of the nipples, together with a heavy, tender feeling of the breasts. These may feel larger very early in pregnancy. The nipples will become harder and are extremely sensitive. They may become browner in colour and small white spots on the areolae may become more pronounced. Breast tenderness usually disappears after about eight weeks of pregnancy.

Taste

You may experience a characteristic taste in your mouth – often described as metallic – and your preferences for food and drinks may change quite markedly, sometimes even before you miss a period.

Pregnant women often go off fried foods, coffee and alcohol (which means that they have no problem resisting them for the sake of their health and that of the baby). They may however have strange new cravings – often cravings that they need to resist if they are for sweet and high-calorie foods, which may be low in nutritional value.

Constipation

This is an irritating fact of pregnancy and contributes to a general sense of bloatedness. It is caused by hormonal changes, making the muscles of the digestive and gastrointestinal systems less efficient than usual.

Do not take any drugs or other remedies for constipation, simply follow the guidelines for a healthy diet described in Eating well and staying in shape, page 62.

147

Your feelings

The baby develops very quickly during the first three months of pregnancy, although little sign of this is apparent to the outside world. In the early months it probably won't even show yet that you are pregnant.

It may seem incredible to you that you are walking around with a tiny miracle developing inside you, yet no one knows about it. You may think that as you feel different you must look different – and yet you don't.

Even by week 12, you probably won't look any different to the outside world. Your uterus is still no bigger than the size of a tennis ball, and so there will hardly be any visible difference in your appearance.

You and your partner will be able to see all sorts of changes, however, when you look at yourself naked in the mirror. Your nipples are probably bigger and the circles around them darker. Your breasts will be fuller and heavier. Yet when you put your clothes back on, no one is any the wiser.

You will also probably feel very different. Your breasts may tingle. You may have a sensation of fullness low in your abdomen. You may want to pass water more often. You may feel slightly sick most of the time. You may feel unusually sleepy at times during the day. Most of the time, however, you probably feel vibrant and excited for now and for the future.

Feeling anxious

Nearly every parent-to-be – and most particularly a mother – experiences some anxieties about their impending role. Will the baby be all right? Will it be normal? What will the birth be like? Will we be good parents? Will we be able to cope?

All these worries are perfectly normal. Many of us experience these feelings during pregnancy. This is not a sign of weakness; it is merely an indication that you are taking your prospective role seriously.

A lot of pregnant women have disturbing dreams about giving birth and about being a mother. Dreams play two important roles. They are, on the one hand, a way of bringing fears to the surface and in this way removing them. They are also a way of "practising" the role you are about to play.

Communicating with your baby

The relationship between the mother and baby is a very special one, and this applies, too, to the days of pregnancy, before the baby is born.

A father may not feel quite as close to the unborn baby as the mother does. This is understandable, as the woman is in immediate and constant physical touch with the growing baby, but it is important for the father to feel involved right from the start.

Some fathers deal with this by enjoying pre-birth "bonding" with their baby by talking to him or her while still in the uterus. There are even fathers who maintain that the baby recognized their voice when he or she was born, presumably because of all those conversations they had in utero. They may be right. No one knows for sure how much a baby sees, hears, feels, or thinks when he or she is in the uterus, but there's certainly no harm in talking to the bump, stroking it, playing it music – whatever appeals to you both.

Your baby's ears are reasonably well formed by the seventh week of pregnancy. It is known that external sounds filter through the mother's abdomen and reach the baby, although they are no doubt changed in quality. The rhythms of these sounds, however, remain unchanged. Ultrasound pictures have shown that a fetus of 24–25 weeks will respond to a noise applied to its mother's abdomen in what is known as a "blink-startle response".

"With sophisticated apparatus," says Dr Leo Simmer, consultant paediatrician and neonatologist at Guy's Hospital in London, "you can show that sending noises through the uterus seems to produce a reaction in the fetus."

It has been shown that unborn babies are not only able to perceive sounds but to remember something about what they heard as well. The baby can recognize intonation patterns: so it is able not just to perceive sounds before it is born, but to learn something about them. The baby may be capable of detecting different speech sounds – such as yours and your partner's.

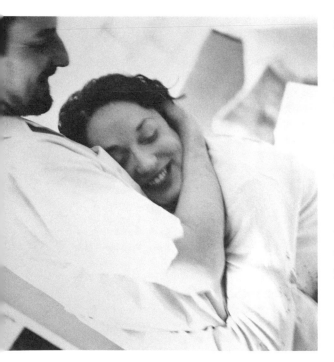

Once your pregnancy is confirmed, you and your partner can look forward to your future as parents, with the bond between you growing even stronger.

149

First 12 weeks of pregnancy

Once you and your partner have received confirmation of your pregnancy – ideally, with the sight of your baby's heartbeat on an ultrasound scan – your thoughts will be alive to the future and the decisions you need to make.

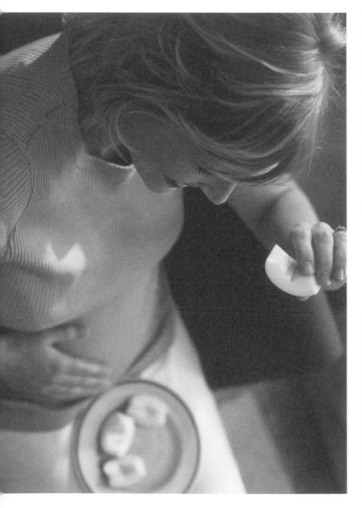

You may want to establish the baby's delivery date with your doctor as soon as you can. The efficient implementation of virtually all diagnostic and therapeutic measures in antenatal care depends on a knowledge of the gestational age, so a scan at about 12 weeks is very important. Medical management of any complications in late pregnancy depends on accurate dating.

You may want to start thinking about what sort of delivery you want – is it to be in hospital

You owe it to yourself and your baby to eat healthily and to get as much rest as you need – and to take time to enjoy these special months of pregnancy.

TIPS FOR A HAPPY, HEALTHY PREGNANCY

- *go to a yoga class for pregnant women*
- *indulge yourself in aromatherapy and massage treatments for aches and pains*
- *take plenty of exercise, especially walking in the fresh air and swimming*
- *take care not to become overtired as it is harder to recover when pregnant*

or at home? Do you wish your partner to be there? Are you thinking of having a water birth?

You may feel irritated by the common conditions associated with pregnancy. The big one is, unsurprisingly, tiredness, but other common conditions include morning sickness,

---

ROUTINE SCREENING TESTS

Once you know that you are pregnant, you will be tested routinely via blood tests for:

- *your blood group (in case you later need a blood transfusion) and to determine whether you are rhesus positive or rhesus negative (see pages 56–7)*

- *your blood count, in case you are anaemic*

- *to check that you are immune to rubella*

- *to check your blood sugar level (done in some units but not others)*

- *to ensure you are free of hepatitis B*

- *to check for HIV if you are in a high risk group or if you ask for the test*

- *to check for signs of sexually transmitted disease, principally gonorrhoea and syphilis*

You will also have a urine test in order to check for kidney disease, diabetes, and urinary tract disease such as cystitis.

---

passing urine nearly non-stop, constipation, haemorrhoids, back ache (always wear flat shoes), and swollen feet. Yet all this is a small price to pay for the new life that you are carrying.

Fatigue and more fatigue

Do everything you can to rest your body and give it the fuel it needs for the developing baby. Eat regularly and well, at least three times a day, preferably more often, and ditch junk food and alcohol. It is better, if you can, to eat five or six smaller meals a day rather than three big ones.

Constipation and morning sickness

Eat plenty of fruit and vegetables and as many wholemeal products as possible. Go for wholemeal bread, wholemeal biscuits, wholemeal pastas, and muesli in order to avoid constipation and haemorrhoids.

Make sure that you drink at least eight glasses of water every day.

Antenatal care

You will receive antenatal care through your family doctor, either at your local hospital or at your family doctor's surgery. Antenatal care in the first three months includes a number of routine screening tests and is intended to identify any possible risk factors.

You will have an antenatal clinic visit at around 12 weeks. An ultrasound scan at this time will confirm the age of the baby, measure its growth, show the baby's heart beating, show any abnormalities, reveal twins (or more), and locate the exact position of the baby should you be having chorionic villus sampling or amniocentesis. In many hospitals, a Down's screening test is offered. This consists of measuring the skin fold on the back of the baby's neck: the nuchal translucency.

Your baby's development

At 3–4 weeks The blastocyst (the term for a fertilized egg with dividing, multiplying cells) implants itself in the lining of the uterus. At this time, your baby is no larger than the size of a single grain of rice and the shape of a tiny seahorse. Nevertheless, the major systems and organs of your baby's body are starting to grow.

At 4–5 weeks The blastocyst is now an embryo. It consists of three layers, from which all its body structures will develop.

At 5–6 weeks Your baby's head is forming. Its heart is beating (and this can be seen on an ultrasound scan at this time), and the legs – no more than tiny buds at first – are growing.

At 6–8 weeks All the baby's internal organs are now in position. The baby is now about 2.5cm (1in) in length.

At 10–11 weeks Your baby is moving about a lot, although you cannot yet feel it. Its eyes are formed. Its fingers and toes are also forming, but they are still joined together by webs of skin.

At 12–13 weeks Your baby is developing at an astonishing rate. Its external genitals are formed, and all its facial features are distinguishable. Its muscles are getting stronger, which means that its movements are getting more vigorous. Ultrasound can pick up the sound of the baby's heartbeat: it is much quicker – twice as fast – than the rate of an adult heartbeat. At 12 weeks, your baby is now some 7.5cm (3in) in length.

Specialized procedures

You may have one or more of the following screening procedures, as well as the routine ones described earlier. You will only have these specialized procedures if you or your baby are perceived to be at risk in any way (see Understanding your fertility, page 12).

Procedure: chorionic villus sampling
When: between weeks 11 and 14
To identify condition: fetal abnormality, hereditary disorder

Procedure: alphafetoprotein blood test
When: between weeks 15 and 22

To identify condition: fetal abnormality, including spinal cord defects

Procedure: amniocentesis
When: between weeks 14 and 20
To identify condition: fetal abnormality, sex of baby

Procedure: cordocentesis (fetal blood sampling)
When: from week 22
To identify condition: rhesus negative mother with antibodies that may destroy baby's blood cells; other genetic conditions

Procedure: ultrasound scan
When: from 18 weeks, certain abnormalities and defects become apparent
To identify condition: defects of spinal cord, abnormalities of head and heart

Exercise

You should take some kind of regular exercise during your pregnancy, preferably every day. The form this takes can be gentle and slow, but it should be regular. Yoga, walking and swimming are all excellent forms of exercise for this period. Warm up first and try not to go for any length of time with no exercise at all. A little each day is better than a lot once in a while.

Exercise assists with both your mental and your physical well-being, because it helps you to relax. It also aids the circulation of your blood, which means that both your body and that of your baby receive plenty of oxygen.

If you stay fit and supple, this will increase the chances of you having an easier labour, as well as making it easier for you to regain your shape after you have given birth.

AVOID THE FOLLOWING:

Don't drink more than six glasses of any alcoholic drink a week • Don't smoke • Don't risk getting overtired

Sleep

The third and very important component of your lifestyle care during pregnancy is sleep.

You will inevitably feel more tired than you usually do – and you will probably be even more tired during the later months of pregnancy. After the delivery of your baby you may face many months of broken nights, and life will be extremely busy.

It is essential therefore to get into the habit, now, of resting when you need to, of getting early nights as a matter of habit, and of listening to your body for the signs of fatigue.

Within a few months, with the delivery of your baby, you will need to feel as refreshed and rested as possible, in order to enjoy the new life you and your partner have created.

153

Finding help

UK
Alcoholics Anonymous
PO Box 1
Stonebow House
Stonebow
York YO1 7NJ
tel: 01904 644026
www.alcoholics-
anonymous.org.uk

Amarant Trust
(for menopause and
premature menopause)
11–13 Charterhouse Buildings
London EC1N 7AN
tel: 020 7401 3855

British Agencies for Adoption
and Fostering
Skyline House
200 Union Street
London SE1 0LX
tel: 020 7593 2000
www.baaf.org.uk

British Diabetic Association
10 Queen Anne Street
London W1M 0BD
tel: 020 7323 1531
www.diabetes.org.uk

CHILD, The National Infertility
Support Network
Charter House
3 St Leonard's Road
Bexhill on Sea
East Sussex TN40 1JA
tel: 01424 732361
www.child.org.uk

Cystic Fibrosis Trust
11 London Road
Bromley
Kent BR1 1BY
tel: 020 8464 7211
www.cftrust.org.uk

Down's Syndrome
Association
155 Mitcham Road
London SW17 9PG
tel: 020 8682 4001
www.downs-syndrome.org.uk

Foresight, The Association for the
Promotion of Preconceptual Care
28 The Paddock
Godalming
Surrey GU7 1XD
tel: 01483 427839

The Human Fertilization and
Embryology Authority
Paxton House
30 Artillery Lane
London E1 7LS
tel: 020 7377 5077
www.hfea.gov.uk/patients
information

Issue/The National Fertility
Association
114 Litchfield Street
Walsall
West Midlands WS1 1SZ
tel: 01922 722888
www.issue.co.uk

Miscarriage Association
Clayton Hospital
Northgate
Wakefield
West Yorkshire WF1 3JS
tel: 01924 200799
www.the-ma.org.uk

Multiple Births Foundation
Queen Charlotte's and Chelsea
Hospital
Goldhawk Road
London W6 0XG
tel: 020 8383 3510
www.multiplebirths.org.uk

National Childbirth Trust
Alexander House
Oldham Terrace
London W3 6NH
tel: 020 8992 8637
www.nct-online.org.uk

National Endometriosis Society
50 Westminster Palace Gardens
1–7 Artillery Row
London SW1P 1RL
tel: 020 7222 2781
www.Endo.org.uk

Quitline (giving up smoking)
helpline: 0800 002200

Relate (relationship counselling)
Herbert Gray College
Little Church Street
Rugby
Warwickshire CV21 3AP
tel: 01788 573241
www.relate.org.uk

Royal College of Obstetricians
and Gynaecologists
27 Sussex Place
London NW1
tel: 020 7772 6200
www.rcog.org.uk

Sickle Cell Society
54 Station Road
London NW10 4UA
tel: 020 8961 4006/7795
www.sicklecellsociety.org.uk

Women's Health
52 Featherstone Street
London EC1Y 8RT
tel: 020 7251 6333
www.womenshealthlondon.org.uk

Women's Healthcare
27a Queen's Terrace
St John's Wood
London NW8 5EA
tel: 020 7483 0099

AUSTRALIA
Australian Council of Natural
Family Planning
PO Box 529
Forestville, NSW 2087
tel/fax (+61) 9452 5244
www.ozemail.com.au/

Maternity Alliance
PO Box 429, Jannali, NSW 2226
tel: 61 3 9348 0249

NEW ZEALAND
Parents Centres NZ Inc
tel: 64 4 560 1990
fax: 64 4 560 1992
www.parentscentre.org.nz

Complementary therapies (UK)

The Institute for Complementary
　Medicine
Tavern Quay
Plough Way
Surrey Quays
London SE16 7QZ
tel: 020 7237 5165

The British Register of
　Complementary Practitioners
Institute for Complementary
　Medicine
PO Box 194
London SE16 7QZ
tel: 020 7237 5165

ACUPUNCTURE
The British Acupuncture Council
63 Jeddo Road
London W12 9HQ
tel: 020 8735 0400

ALEXANDER TECHNIQUE
The Society of Teachers of the
　Alexander Technique
129 Camden Mews
London
NW1 9AH
tel: 020 7284 3338
www.stat.org.uk

AROMATHERAPY
The International Federation of
　Aromatherapists
182 Chiswick High Rd
London W4 1PP
tel: 020 8742 2605

HERBALISM
The National Institute of
　Medical Herbalists
9 Palace Gate
Exeter EX1 1JA
tel: 01392 426022

Bach Flower Remedies
Bach Centre
Mount Vernon
Sotwell

Wallingford
Oxon OX10 0PZ
tel: 01491 839489

HOMEOPATHY
The British Homeopathic
　Association
15 Clerkenwell Close
London EC1R 0AA
tel: 020 7566 7800

HYPNOTHERAPY
The British Hypnotherapy
　Association
1 Wythburn Place
London W1H 5WL
tel: 020 7723 4443

The British Society for Medical
　and Dental Hypnosis
4 Kirkwood Avenue
Cookridge
Leeds LS16 7JU
tel: 0113 2857768

MASSAGE
The London College of Massage
5 Newman Passage
London W1P 3PN
tel: 020 7323 3574

MEDITATION
If you would like to join a group to
learn how to meditate, you may
find a list in your local library, or
they may advertise in your local
paper or in health food shops.
Alternatively, contact the
following:

School of Meditation
158 Holland Park Avenue
London W11 4UH
tel: 020 7603 6116

OSTEOPATHY
The General Osteopathic Council
Osteopathy House
176 Tower Bridge Road
London SE1 3LU
tel: 020 7357 6655

REFLEXOLOGY
The Association of Reflexologists
27 Old Gloucester Street
London WC1N 3XX
tel: 0870 5673320

VISUALIZATION THERAPY
Therapists who frequently use
visualization include
psychotherapists and
hypnotherapists, as well as
specialists in biofeedback,
autogenic training, and rebirthing.

YOGA
British Wheel of Yoga
25 Jermyn Street
Sleaford
Lincolnshire NG34 7RU
tel: 01529 306851

The Iyengar Yoga Institute
223a Randolph Avenue
London W9 1NL
tel: 020 7624 3080

Further reading

Belinda Barnes and Suzanne Gail Bradley in association with Foresight, The Association for The Promotion of Preconceptual Care: *Planning for a Healthy Baby* (Vermilion, 1990)

Hilary Boyd: *Working Woman's Pregnancy* (Mitchell Beazley, 2001)

Anne Charlish: *A Woman's Guide to Birth-Tech: Tests and Technology in Pregnancy and Birth* (Christopher Helm, 1989)

Anne Charlish: *Your Natural Baby: Complementary Therapies for the First Three Years* (Connections 1996)

Anne Charlish: *Your Natural Pregnancy: A Guide to Complementary Therapies* (Boxtree, 1995)

Glade B Curtis, MD, FACOG: *Your Pregnancy Over 30* (Element, 1998)

Marilyn Glenville: *Natural Solutions to Infertility* (Piatkus, 2000)

Harriet Griffey: *How to Get Pregnant* (Bloomsbury, 1997)

Maggie Jones: *Infertility: Modern Treatments and the Issues they Raise* (Piatkus, 1991)

Sally Keeble: *Conceiving Your Baby: How Medicine Can Help* (Cedar/Mandarin, 1995)

Dr Mary Ann Lumsden et al: *Royal College of Obstetricians and Gynaecologists/Complete Women's Health* (Thorsons, 2000)

Dr Ann Robinson: *The Which? Guide to Women's Health* (Which? Books, 1999)

Sherman J Silber, MD: *How to get Pregnant with the New Technology* (Warner Books, 1998)

Allan Templeton et al: *Management of Infertility for the MRCOG and Beyond* (RCOG Press, 2000)

Professor Robert Winston, MB, BS, FRCOG: *Getting Pregnant: The Complete Guide to Fertility and Infertility* (Pan, 1989)

Professor Robert Winston, MB, BS, FRCOG: *Infertility: A Sympathetic Approach* (Martin Dunitz, 1986)

156

Index

159

Acknowledgements

I am greatly indebted to Dr Donald Gibb for his diligence and humour as consultant for this book. I am also indebted to Professor Gedis Grudzinskas and Patricia Roberts for their assistance on the subjects of infertility and pregnancy. I am grateful to Mr Malcolm Whitehead for his insights into the menopause and premature menopause. Lastly, I am greatly indebted to Professor Robert Winston for his tireless research and illuminating publications into the complex subject of infertility.

Picture credits

2–3 Image Bank/Tom Mareschal; 9 Stone/James McEntee; 13 Science Photo Library/Phil Jude; 25 Photodisc; 26 Science Photo Library/James Stevenson; 31 Stone/Martin Barraud; 33 Image State; 39 Science Photo Library/Adam Hart-Davis; 44 Science Photo Library/D. Phillips; 47 Science Photo Library; 51 Stone/Stefan May; 59 Stone/Colin Barker; 63 Stone/Erik Dreyer; 65 Stone/Adamski Peek; 70 Image State; 72 Octopus Publishing Group Ltd/Hamlyn/David Jordan; 74 Image State; 79 Photodisc; 83 Stone/Philip & Karen Smith; 96 Stone/Kaz Chiba; 100 AKG, London; 103 Powerstock Zefa/Wickenthey; 106 Photodisc; 110 Stone/Chris Craymer; 117 Science Photo Library/Cordelia Molloy; 119 Octopus Publishing Group Ltd/Mitchell Beazley/Kevin Summers; 121 Image Bank/Piecework Productions; 125 Stone/Paul Arthur; 128 Octopus Publishing Group Ltd/Hamlyn/Mark Winwood; 133 Pictor International; 139 Science Photo Library/Philippe Plailly/Eurelios; 140 Stone/Clarissa Leahy; 143 Mother & Baby Picture Library/Paul Mitchell; 145 Stone/Stuart McClymont; 149 Stone/Victoria Yee; 150 Stone/Ian O'Leary